MEDICINE
THAT
KILLS

French edition of this book "Des Médicaments qui tuent" First published in 1998 by:

Louise Courteau, Éditrice inc.
481, Chemin du Lac-Saint-Louis Est
Saint-Zénon (Québec) Canada
J0K 3N0

Canadian Cataloguing in Publication Data

Kolp, Viviane, 1957-
    Medicine that kills

    Translation of: Des médicaments qui tuent.
    Includes bibliographical references.
    ISBN 0-9680085-2-6

    1. Scheuer, Yvette – Health. 2. Medicine, Botanic – Case studies. 3. Alternative medicine – Case studies. 4. Therapeutics, Physiological – Case studies. I. Title.

RV8.S33K6613 1999   615.5'3'092   C98-901297-2

Cover design by: Guy Ledoux

Text design by: CompoMagny enr.

Printed and bound in Canada by: Transcontinental printing

Distributed by: Hushion House publishing limited

MEDICINE THAT KILLS

Viviane Kolp,
with the collaboration
of Yvette Scheuer

Also by Viviane Kolp

The Love of Life (Poetry)
Medicine that kills
Once upon a remedy

*This book is
dedicated to
my mother
and to
the future*

Acknowledgments

I wish to express my deep and lasting appreciation to my sister Chantal for having assisted mother and me in the preparation of this book, as well as our friend Teresa Zahorodna, B.A., LL.B. for her encouragement and help in editing. We also wish to acknowledge my brothers Robert and Gerry as well as my sister Brigitte for their help.

Our very special thanks go to my mother's brother Joseph (Josy) for his reliable help in editing the french edition of this book.

Important, please read

The information in this book is intended to increase your awareness of preventive health care. By no means is it intended to diagnose or treat your medical problem or ailment. The regimens throughout this book are recommendations, not prescriptions, and are not intended as medical advice. Any decision you make, involving the treatment of your illness is your responsibility and should include the guidance of either a medical doctor of your choice or a professional health counselor, especially if you have a specific physical problem or are taking any medication.

About the Author

Viviane Kolp was born in Arlon, Belgium, a little town only steps away from Luxembourg. She is the fourth of eight children, four brothers and three sisters.

Her family emigrated to Canada in 1969. They lived in Montreal until their move to Vancouver in 1978. Her father passed away in 1986.

Her languages include: French, English, Luxembourg (dialect) and German. She has attended classical ballet school from early childhood until early adulthood.

She holds a diploma in Modern Massage, certificates in Practical Massage, Human Anatomy & Physiology, Medical Terminology, Psychology & Social Work, and is a certified Pharmaceutical Assistant.

She has worked as an independent massage therapist for the past twenty years, the last fifteen of which in private practice.

Viviane lives with her mother who is her greatest supporter. They have a very special and close relationship. It is for her she writes this book, she also writes to share with others an awareness of the healing powers of natural remedies that are often overlooked, even when conventional medicine fails. After all, nature is a most needed resource and even science cannot surpass its powers!

Table of Contents

Introduction

This book has been written to illustrate how love of one's fellow man and woman can have a powerful therapeutic and healing effect. Love is the most amazing emotion and one that refuses to accept most accepted wisdoms.

Love makes us question accepted knowledge, especially when that knowledge fails to cure or alleviate the pain and suffering of a loved one. This love also calls into question the infallibility of the medical system and medical practitioners who administer the system.

It is a known fact that in most professions familiarity breeds an acceptance of establishment operating procedures even when time and again such methods are proven to have results other than those anticipated. Witness the huge number of malpractice suits filed each year. The human body and the human psyche are so individualized that any one procedure, no matter how well accepted, cannot be expected to work for each person. Additionally, medical science is turning up many, many new ailments and a corresponding number of variations of known diseases and medical conditions.

The love of a daughter for her mother is often so powerful that it has the effect of bypassing normal medical practices and performing what could only be called miracles.

With medicine being such an inexact science it is not surprising that confusion can occur. Medicine which may have a healing effect on one person with a known disease will not have the same effect on another person with what has been diagnosed as the same disease. Each person reacts differently to drugs, pills, diets and medications. This often leads to the cure being worse than the supposed disease and results in ongoing pain and despair in the victim.

In my mother's case it was the endless years of being on prescription medicine that led to what is medically known as Fatty Liver Infiltration, which becomes fatal unless measures are taken to eliminate the cause. For mother that was impossible because only pescribed pain killers could alleviate the severity of her chronic headaches.

For starters, you should know that in the long run all medication, whether over the counter or prescribed, will cause you serious and sometimes irreparable damage due to its side effects. Drug therapy takes an immense toll on the human body and could contribute to an early demise. Medications deal primarily with symptoms and are basically used to help control some complications, not cure them. Many drugs interact with one another and that is when side effects occur.

This is what was happening to my mother, in one way or another, for almost three years. During that time period she also developed what was said to be an allergy, affecting her face and buttock area, giving the appearance of a third degree burn. Because her physician was unable to diagnose the condition or to determine the cause, it was left unattended. It wasn't until several months later, through our continuous research of medical and natural healing books and the ongoing insistence for more blood tests, that we were able to learn that the cause was due to undetected diabetes mellitus.

The diabetes was a drawback as it entailed taking more medication, which adversely affected her already deteriorating liver. Since treatments vary so widely among medical professionals, no single approach proved to be ideal for mother and further opinions were always needed. We finally gave up on the doctors' unproven theories and simply followed our own.

My instincts told me to undertake reading the medical dictionary as fast as I could to try to find what the doctors perhaps overlooked. Time was as big an enemy as was mother's illness. Thank heaven I found the answer to the liver problem in the first half of my research. It actually overwhelmed me to find out that the particular remedy completely reverses fatty liver infiltration as well as numerous other conditions.

Why is it that doctors won't supply this cure? The reason they don't is because it is only available as a natural supplement, and as such, against the beliefs of conventional medical practitioners. I purchased a bottle of it and within two days, mother improved dramatically and is continuing to do so. It also worked on her diabetic problem and she is now free of her medication.

We are very grateful to and respect nature, for it protects us in more ways than one. Regardless of how strong science may be, it shall never defeat the powers of nature. We have not been created just to fill up space, to think that way would be an eternal shame. All of us have special talents, certain understandings and in a sense it becomes our personal obligation to help other human beings in any way we can. It has nothing to do with power, it has to do with loving and being concerned about other human conditions. We feel it is our duty to share and make visible what is unseen and what is misinformed, if informed at all.

Take our parents for example, they are now starting to pass away, some of them much too soon. Even though the flame is passed on, this flame has become very weak. It needs to be re-ignited. Please don't let it extinguish.

P.S.

The natural remedies are the secret to this book! Our success story is not to be swept aside for the failure of conventional medicine. That is why the actual pictures and laboratory test results are included as proof.

CHAPTER I

Mother, The Early Years

A FRAGILE BEGINNING

On a beautiful spring day in March, 1932, in Luxembourg, one of the most splendid and tiniest Countries in this world, what should have been a blessing, turned rapidly into a tragedy. My mother was born to an identical twin brother and neither of them was expected to survive due to their lack of weight. It was a daily battle just trying to keep them alive. My mother had one extra pound to her advantage, which ended up saving her life, while her twin sadly lost his fight for dear life just three months later.

Even though my mother survived, her frail state kept her parents in a continuous state of distress, fearful of losing her as well. Her mother wasn't willing to experience another loss and therefore provided her with the best medicine of all "an abundant amount of motherly love and comfort", which comes instinctively towards the one or ones you wish to protect and love unconditionally!

As time went by, my mother gained strength, but fatigue started taking a toll on her mother's health. My grandmother was only twenty-six years of age and expecting, any day, the birth of her sixth child. Fortunately, she could always depend on her ever supportive brother, my great-uncle Albert, who, although a bachelor, was always willing to lend his assistance in times of need.

It wasn't long before the arrival of my mother's healthy baby sister was announced. But the same thing could not be said for my grandmother who did not appear to be recovering from the birth as well as would be expected. It was then that the midwife in all sincerity proposed to care for the new little baby girl for as long as it would require my grandmother to get well. The idea was gratefully accepted.

Three weeks later, on a piercing cold November morning, my grandmother was re-admitted to the hospital. On the way to the hospital, as if she had a premonition, my grandmother asked her brother Albert to stop at a photography studio for a portrait, which proved to be the only picture that her children would ever have to remember her by.

From that day onward everything just crumbled. A week later, my grandmother tragically died, supposedly from an internal infection, leaving behind her six young children, five girls and one boy, ranging in ages from eight years to three weeks.

Even before the funeral took place, my grandfather made the hasty decision to place his children in an orphanage in the expectation that they would receive a good education and would grow up within sight of each other. He was totally opposed to the persistent but kind offers to care for the children from several close family members who were themselves childless and financially comfortable. Many years later, my grandfather came to bitterly regret his decision.

In the years that followed, my mother and her brother and sisters seldom saw their father as he was being treated, off and on, for depression brought on by the passing of his beloved wife.

My mother's uncle Albert kept putting on a brave face even though he was heartbroken in more ways than one.

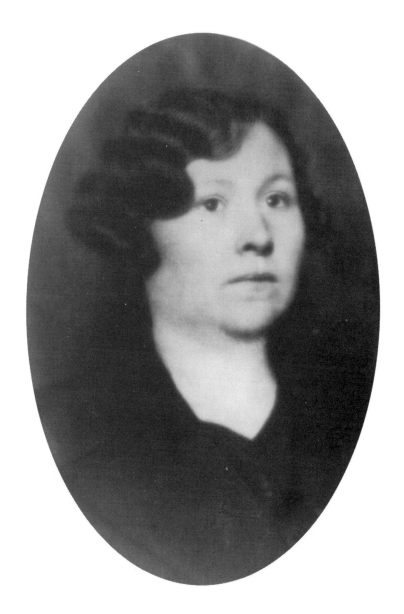

LOUISE FLENER

My mother's mother at the age of 26,
several days before her death.
She was survived by her six children ages three weeks
to eight years.

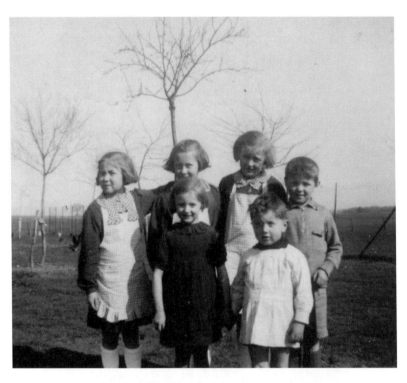

From center counter-clockwise, my mother with
her cousin YVAN, brother JOSEPH, and sisters
CÉCILE, GERMAINE and ROSY.

Not only did he live with the grief of having just lost his sister at so young an age, but also the restriction of limited access to her six children whom he loved as dearly as if they were his own. Never could he pardon my grandfather for having committed the children to an orphanage. In the four years the children were confined to the orphanage, great-uncle Albert never missed a Sunday visit with them.

Many years later my great-uncle Albert would recall to my mother the desolation he felt when he saw his nieces and nephew on his first visit to the orphanage. He had stood in complete disbelief when he saw that his nieces' beautiful long locks had been shorn, and that his nephew had also been subjected to the ruthless hands of a barber. The boy's bare head only emphasized the dejection in his upturned face. The fence dividing the boys' section at the orphanage allowed little contact with the boy's sisters, so what little contact he did have at recess became the highlight of his day.

The first year at the orphanage had a considerable impact on all of the children because they were deprived of the maternal love which had been so cruelly taken away from them at an age when they needed it most. Mother's health was again poor.

Four years had passed and the children had somewhat adjusted to the generalized style of institution life. The only joyful time for them was the Sunday visits with their uncle Albert.

One startling day their seldom-seen father appeared before them accompanied by an unknown woman who was formally introduced to them as their future new mother. The children responded spontaneously with mistrust and took a couple of steps backwards. After a few moments of stunned silence, enormous tears started rolling down their little innocent faces. The two eldest replied defensively,

"This woman in not our mother!". Being older, they had perfect recollections of their natural mother and were not about to welcome a replacement. To them, the woman was an enemy.

Suffering the loss of a parent is a great pain for a young child, as grief strikes him in the same way it does an adult. It would be unjust to think that because a child is young, he fails to remember. The death of a loved one also means that a part of him will be forever gone. It's a change that brings grief and is not as cut and dried as it may seem. Although the grief fades, the hurt remains a constant shadow that forever accompanies him wherever he goes.

Grief has several stages from denial to acceptance, but will be particularly acute in the years immediately following the loss. For children, parents are precious for they are their utmost connection to the past and the greatest influence on their future.

To change what had now become the children's way of life would further deepen their wounds at a time when they were valiantly attempting to cope with their painful past. They had been deprived of a companion and undoubtedly missed their mother's physical presence. They had little choice however when two weeks later they were picked up from the orphanage to embark on a life marked by years of cold rejection and regular beatings by their step-mother while their father was absent. It became a living hell!

HAPPINESS WITH UNCLE ALBERT

Several months went by when my great-uncle Albert approached my grandfather and proposed taking my mother to live with him and his mother. As my mother was showing signs of increasing ill health, my grandfather accepted the proposition.

My mother knew she would miss her brother and sisters when she left, but nothing prepared her for the pain and sadness that gripped her upon the realization that for the others, there would be no early escape from the mistreatment they endured.

The two years my mother lived with her uncle Albert were the most memorable ones for her. The love and comfort she received were comparable to what she received from her own mother. Regrettably, it was not enough to avoid her bout with anemia and regular nose bleeds, accompanied by periodic headaches which were bad enough to miss occasional school days. She saw a doctor on a monthly basis.

At that time there was nothing available other than good nutrition and a serene environment which, over time, contributed to a satisfactory return to health for my mother. Her prospect for the future looked bright until one day, in May of 1940, she was awakened by her grandmother's scream. Her grandmother quickly told her to rush downstairs as she could see, looking down from a tiny window, my grandfather coming to retrieve his daughter.

Within minutes of his arrival, my grandfather explained that he was taking his daughter because the Germans were about to divide Belgium from Luxembourg and he would no longer be allowed to visit.

My great-uncle Albert was called to duty by the Belgian military so his mother was left alone in her house.

THE EVIL STEP-MOTHER

When my mother was reunited with her brother and sisters, she had to quickly readjust to the dreadful life she had left behind two years earlier. She had acquired two new step-sisters in the meantime, who were denied nothing,

25

while my mother was denied the affection she had grown to cherish.

Her step-mother would repeatedly inflict retribution on my mother and my aunt. As punishment, her step-mother would immerse my mother's head under ice-cold running tap water. The children would be threatened with worse beatings if they dared to mention their treatment to their father, who was often away from home. As a result, my mother's health deteriorated.

Several years passed before my mother was seen by a doctor. The doctor recommended placing my mother in a specialized care centre for children to conduct tests to determine the cause of her severe headaches. My grandfather was in the process of admitting my mother to the children's care centre when they announced that they were no longer accepting new patients due to the continuous political strife of War.

While my grandfather was weak and recovering from a bout with pneumonia, his wife, who was of German origin, fled with the children and sought refuge in Germany. Due to the number of people seeking refuge in Germany, there were no accommodations for the entire family so the children were dispersed and taken into the homes of various German families. The children were glad to escape the authority of their "evil step-mother". They preferred the continuous aerial bombardment to her tyranny, and lived the last year of the War in relative contentment despite the nightly attacks, the destruction and the American invasion of Germany.

While living with a German family, my mother was afraid to mention her ill health for fear of being returned to the custody of her step-mother. In silence, she endured her headaches which had become much worse. She became aware that certain odors would trigger her attacks. She dreaded going down to the kitchen on Friday mornings, as she could smell the wine sauce that would be simmering for the fish to be served at lunch time. She often ran unnoticed to the bathroom to be sick. On those days she tried to disappear from the house without being seen or missed.

In 1945 when the War ended, all citizens of Luxembourg who had fled to Germany were warned to return to their home country. Upon the family's arrival at the Luxembourg train station, my grandfather and his wife were taken into custody for conspiring with the Germans. It was a scene of utter chaos. Many persons were being arrested while crying children desperately tried to cling to their parents. People were being thrown into military trucks and driven away to various institutions already overcrowded with political prisoners. My mother, her brother and younger sister were sent to one institution, while her three older sisters were sent to a prison camp where they would end up spending two years.

For the next two months, my great-uncle Albert and his mother, who were both Belgian citizens, desperately tried to keep track of the whereabouts of the children. After proving their relationship to the children, and complying with numerous formalities, they were able to get my mother out of the institution. You can imagine how thrilled she was to be removed to a peaceful environment.

A few weeks later, just as it seemed that things were returning to normal, my mother was found one morning limp as a rag doll, with a raging fever and unable to take any nourishment. Upon examination the doctor suspected a recurrence of anemia and immediately administered a shot of penicillin. The next twelve hours were critical. Great-uncle Albert was so concerned with my mother's rapid deterioration that he sped off on his motorcycle to a nearby village to summon a priest to administer the last rights. My mother was not expected to recover and spent the night in a semi-comatose state while her uncle Albert and his mother kept a constant vigil over her.

At the crack of dawn my mother appeared to miraculously come around and the worst was over. She was bedridden for two weeks and was only allowed to get up for one hour a day. After three months, the doctor finally gave permission for her to return to school.

Things seemed to settle down into a normal routine for my mother except for the constant recurring headaches which had been diagnosed as genetically transmitted from the paternal side of her family. No medicine or treatment was available at the time, but the doctors hoped that with time, my mother would outgrow her condition.

Not long after my mother's fifteenth birthday, her stepmother reappeared in her life. As my mother looked strong enough to obtain employment, her step-mother insisted that it was her duty to contribute to the costly medical expenses for the care of her step-sister, who was afflicted with polio.

For the next two years the children worked and their step-mother collected their monthly wages from them. On my mother's eighteenth birthday, her brother and sisters all decided that they would no longer satisfy their step-mother's demands and each prepared to venture forth in separate directions. Except on rare occasions, they never saw their step-mother again.

MOTHER FINDS FREEDOM

My mother found employment as a chambermaid at a small hotel across from the train station in Arlon, Belgium. A tiny room and meals made up for the modest income and long hours of work. She was happy, and for the first time in her life, could do as she pleased with her money.

She distinctly remembers purchasing her first lipstick, a wallet and a small purse to hold what little personal possesions she had. It came to her notice that young men seemed attracted to her and it felt good to receive a different kind of attention.

This new-found freedom served to strengthen my mother's timid personality. On the weekends she rode the train to visit her uncle Albert who was now married and had one son. Her grandmother Annie marvelled at my mother's strength of character and maturity.

During the winter months my mother and her uncle attended the Sunday live theatre performances. It was during one such performance that she noticed a tall, dark and handsome Clark Gable look-alike, who, when he noticed her glances, gestured that he would like to take her to the dance that followed the play. After some gentle persuasion, my great-uncle Albert agreed that she could spend a half hour with the young man at the dance.

Needless to say, my mother and the gentleman, called Roger, enjoyed every precious minute they spent together on the dance floor. When my mother revealed that she worked opposite the train station, Roger was ecstatic, as he worked close by. He was a tailor by trade and reputed to be one of the best.

I am told that Roger tended to indulge in Belgian pastries and french fries, and frivolously spent his money on every movie that ever came out. Luckily for him, he had a metabolism that allowed him to eat anything he pleased without ever gaining a pound. He was tall, measuring six feet one inch, and weighed eighty to eighty-five kilos. In contrast, my mother was petite, standing five feet two inches, and gracefully thin at fifty to fifty-five kilos.

After a nine month courtship, Roger proposed marriage. Great-uncle Albert and his mother had some reservation about the union, as Roger's nonchalant manner gave the appearance that he was not yet ready for the responsibility of marriage. My mother married Roger in October of 1950 and moved to the countryside.

MARRIED LIFE

My parents' first year and a half of marriage was filled with joy and bright ideas for the future. My father was reluctant to have children as he felt children would be in the way and would diminish the attention that he himself craved. My mother did not share in his opinion and planned to have children in the not too distant future.

In the summer of 1951, my mother received a surprise visit from her eldest sister and her husband. They enjoyed a pleasant afternoon together trading stories about past and present events. The sisters made a promise that whichever one of them became pregnant first, the other would stand as godmother to the child.

My mother was greatly affected by her sister's desire for children. She knew her sister suffered from heart disease and had grave doubts about her having children. In December of that year, my mother and her sister exchanged holiday wishes and planned for a visit in the spring. My mother concealed from her sister the fact that she was pregnant as she wished to surprise her in the spring.

One week into January of 1952, my mother received a telegram dreadfully informing her of her sister's sudden death. Her sister had been only twenty-six. The whole family was devastated.

Time seemed to drag on for my mother. In her fourth month of pregnancy she went for her first consultation with an obstetrician. The doctor did not seem as pleased as would have been expected, but all he said at that time was that my mother did not have the physical strength and was not meant to bear children.

In the summer of 1952, after a lengthy and difficult home birth assisted by only a midwife, my mother gave birth to a healthy baby girl. My father did not seem displeased, but neither did he wish to have an input in the care of the child. He went about his daily routine as if nothing had changed.

Mother, on the other hand, was greatly pleased with her little bundle of joy and delighted in playing the role of full-time housewife and mom.

Six months later, after regaining her strength and having adapted to motherhood, she woke up one morning with a familiar symptom which brought her abruptly out of bed.

Mother did not look forward to her appointment with the obstetrician who would not, from a medical point of view, be pleased about her second pregnancy. The doctor refused to disclose the reason for his disapproval, only informing my mother of the danger of miscarriage. She was annoyed with the doctor's opinion and, upon returning home, did not chose to share his opinion with my father. She determined to take extra good care of herself just to prove the doctor wrong.

To the doctor's great surprise, she gave birth to a beautiul baby boy in December of 1953. The attending midwife did need to call for the doctor's assistance during the birth. That is when the doctor told her that my mother should never again be permitted to have a home delivery. He continued to stand firm in his opinion that my mother was at high risk and in future would require professional medical attention. Again he counselled my mother not to attempt to have any more children.

As 1955 came along, my mother again found herself in an interesting condition. Having taken seriously her doctor's advice, she insisted on moving to the city where medical assistance was more accessible. It turned out to be the right decision as she did need medical assistance when in October she delivered an eleven pound baby boy.

Two years later (almost like clockwork), she gave birth to me. Mother was very happy about my arrival as now she felt her family was even, with two boys and two girls. What was troubling my mother, and which she grew to despise in my father, was his constant tendency to move. He was never content living in the same place for long and always felt the need to seek what he thought were greener pastures.

Mother was beginning to be fed up with father's desire to move and on occasion, had to insist firmly that he be patient as she did not like having to take us children out of school before the school year ended.

MOTHER'S CRISIS

In February of 1959, my mother was again expecting to give birth any day. At 4:00 o'clock in the morning she awoke, and upon rising felt so faint that she fell back upon the bed. She knew that something was definitely wrong. She turned on the light and tried to wake up my sleeping father. It took a few seconds to get his attention as he was by now used to being a father and was not overly alarmed that the baby was coming. Only after my mother told him that she was hemorrhaging did he get up in a panic.

There was no telephone in the house and my father decided to go to the nearest public telephone, about one kilometer away. The next-door neighbours had a telephone but my father preferred not to disturb them that early in the morning.

Until my father could return with an ambulance, mother lay as still as she could so as not to aggravate what was already a critical situation. She endured excruciating pain and got terribly frightned upon seeing a large puddle of blood accumulating at the side of the bed. Mother felt the baby inside her kicking desperately. After a while, those powerful little kicks became less and less frequent and eventually stopped entirely.

My mother knew in her heart that the baby had given up its fight for life. She was hoping to hang on until help arrived, but as the minutes crept on she became increasingly alarmed at the thought that my father had managed to get lost. The little clock on the night stand showed almost six a.m. so my father had been gone for two hours.

My mother sensed the strangeness of the quiet house in which her children were still sleeping peacefully. Soon, she knew, the children would be hungry. She prayed to God that they would not come into her room and see their mother in a pool of blood. As she felt herself slipping away she heard the faint sound of a distant siren.

My mother remembers how, on her way to the hospital, the ambulance attendant gently but persistently patted her hand and encouraged her to stay awake. Her last recollection was being wheeled into the emergency room and hearing the doctors and nurses talking about preparing her for a cesarean section. She recalls vaguely hearing one of the doctor's mentioning that the baby had not survived.

A very important detail I must mention is that the reason mother did not hemorrhage to death was because she unconsciously assumed a semi-fetal position which forced the baby's weight to fall on one side generating enough pressure to temporarily stem blood flow.

Mother was in surgery for well over three hours. Father was sent home and told to return in a few hours to answer questions about why it took such unconscionably long time for him to get medical assistance.

Father later explained that when he got to the phone booth the phone was out-of-order so he went to the residence of a prominent obstetrician for help. When he rung the doorbell, a very disgruntled servant leaned out the window and asked him if my mother was the doctor's patient. Upon being informed that my mother was not a patient, the servant told my father not to bother waiting for the doctor as she had strict instructions never to disturb the doctor unless it involved one of his patients.

It is difficult for me to understand why neither my father nor the servant had the presence of mind to call an ambulance from the doctor's house. Mind you, my father never had been very resourceful, perhaps due to the meningitis he had contracted as a young child.

In any case, following his encounter with the servant, father became panicked and disoriented for some time as he walked aimlessly looking for help. He accosted a passer-by and asked for assistance. Dumbfounded, the stranger replied "But sir, you are within steps of the police station! Go ahead and they'll get all the help you need".

By now utterly exhausted, my father staggered to the police station. The Gendarme, after hearing a brief explanation, promptly made the necessary arrangements to rush help to my mother. My father, while fervently hoping and praying that his wife was still alive, was being lectured by the Gendarme about taking three hours to get help when the situation could have been resolved in twenty minutes.

The doctors ultimately accepted father's explanation after questioning the servant who had refused to rouse her employer for the medical emergency. The hospital intended to investigate the obstetrician for medical negligence.

Finally, after what seemed to be an endless interrogation, my father was told about the loss of the baby. The baby was a nine and half pound boy. As for my mother's condition, the doctors said it would take another twenty-four hours before they could determine if she was out of danger. My father was allowed to see her for only a few minutes.

For three days mother remained under constant supervision in the intensive-care unit. The hospital, being a catholic hospital, was managed by a religious order of nuns who took excellent care of her.

As mother was on a liquid diet, the nun in charge prepared her own recipe which she truly believed in and had administered successfully to other patients.

THE COGNAC/EGG ENERGY RECIPE

She blended two ounces of French cognac with one egg and two tablespoons of sugar and fed the mixture to my mother for breakfast. She recommended that my mother continue drinking this potion for six weeks after returning home from the hospital and to make use of it at anytime she felt her strength waning.

To this day we still use this remedy, particularly in the winter months when flu bugs are rampant.

UNCLE ALBERT DIES

A week after this crisis, mother was gratefully back home with all of us. She considered herself doubly blessed, because I, being the littlest one at sixteen months, never cried or made a fuss. I cuddled up to my mother as though I sensed the pain she was in and was trying to comfort her.

Around this time my mother received an unexpected visit from her brother. He had just received a letter advising of uncle Albert's death and had come on the unpleasant task of informing my mother of the death of their beloved uncle Albert at the age of forty-two.

My great-uncle Albert had been admitted to the hospital with pneumonia at the same time as my mother had been admitted to Emergency. Neither one was aware of the other's sudden medical crisis.

There are no words to describe the profound pain the news brought to my mother especially as she did not even have the opportunity to attend his funeral to pay her last respects.

My great-uncle Albert was a very special man who had a profound effect on my mother's upbringing. He gave her the only happiness she knew as a young child. His memory merits living on. It is my reason for having written this poem.

Dealing with these back-to-back distressful incidents demanded a great deal of bravery on my mother's part. Despite the hurt she had sustained, she had to put aside her grief as her first responsibility was first and foremost to her children.

To protect her health and ensure the children's futures, she made the difficult decision to request her doctor to perform a tubal ligation. Inexplicably, since the doctor had always insisted that my mother not have any more children, he refused to perform the procedure.

In Memory
of
My Mother's Uncle Albert

He was young, he was strong,
and for a while
to her he did belong.
Their time has come and gone.
His death she had to overcome,
even though a lasting grief
had just begun.
Much too soon
this loving being was taken away
and now and again
she looks up at the moon
dreaming of the days
when they used to play.
As a young child
she was at times a little wild,
but he never did mind
because he was so very kind.
Many days were spent with him
at her grandma's place,
and she'll always remember
his happy face.
How she misses his shiny motorbike,
just as she wishes
they could go
for another country hike.
He had his ways to chase away
one's scariest moments,
and he always knew how to erase
even the littlest of torments.
Together they were quite a pair
and forever she'll remember
what they once did share.
To her he was the dearest man.
She was his greatest fan.

My mother became angry and demanded some answers from the doctor. He had no choice but to reveal the cause of his concern. He informed her that as her blood type was A-Negative and my father's blood type was O-Positive, each pregnancy posed a danger to her and the unborn child.

Today, this condition is no longer a worry as long as your physician is aware of it. In mother's day, however, her obstetrician had seldom seen women in that condition carry a child to term. And those women who did took the risk that their children could be afflicted with Downs Syndrome, a congenital defect usually caused by the presence of an extra No. 21 chromosome (trisomy) characterized by mental retardation.

Upon hearing this news, mother was speechless. She thanked her lucky stars that all her chidlren turned out to be healthy, beautiful babies. The doctor suggested that my mother try contraceptives, and she agreed to give it a try. Disappointingly, my mother had to stop taking contraceptives three months later as her system simply could not tolerate them.

It appeared as though any unnatural substance worked against my mother's physiological state. Even the prescription medication for her ongoing headaches produced unpleasant side effects and she refused to be on any medication as she was pregnant every other year. She tried to control the pain of her annoying headaches through self-control and by focussing her attention on her children.

Her deliverance from pain would not come about for a long time as between 1959 and 1967 she had four more babies. In the end, my mother had four girls and four boys. She had such difficulties with her last two pregnancies that her doctor believed that she would not survive another pregnancy and gave his permission for a tubal ligation. After all those years, she thought she would finally have peace of mind.

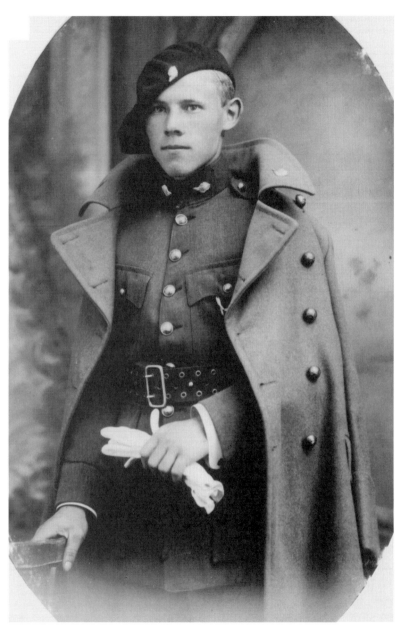

ALBERT FLENER
My mother's uncle

Chapter II

Coming to Canada

Father makes a startling announcement

In September, 1968, father announced that he had a big surprise, and what a big surprise it turned out to be!

Mother was shocked to learn that without her knowledge or consent, father had obtained a passport, withdrew all the money from their bank account and was leaving for Canada in two days! He wanted to check out the possibilities for a more advantageous future in Canada. If all worked out as planned, the family could join him at a later date. My father excitedly said, "Wish me good luck. Montreal, here I come!".

Mother was furious as she felt that my father was trying to act like a bachelor free of responsibility for his family. She was left to run the business which sold exclusive and made-to-measure men's wear. She juggled her work at the store as well as take care of eight children without a baby-sitter.

The heavy load of responsibilities took a toll on her health and soon after she was advised that she had to have a dilatation and curettage (D and C) to stop the heavy bleeding which came on abruptly.

At the hospital, the doctor also told her that a hysterectomy (surgical removal of the uterus) was unavoidable if the condition showed no improvement. Mother was against the idea and put off making a decision until it became necessary. She felt she could not permit herself to stay in the hospital for any period of time because there was no one to look after us children. She released herself from the hospital, promising to rest at home until she was capable of going about her duties.

Fortunately, my older sister and brother were a great help to her while she was recuperating at home. We were all so close to our mother and received so much love from her that we did not let her out of our sight. It was not a difficult task to look out for one another as we were all well behaved, calm, and well disciplined children.

While these events were occuring, father, according to his letters to us, was on cloud nine in Montreal. In his letters he painted a completely different picture from the one we saw upon our arrival eight months later. Home turned out to be a tourist house where father had rented one large room for the entire family, which he said would have to do until he could afford a larger place.

We could see that father had acquired a new free style and irresponsible attitude. We became distant and resentful. Mother cried. We children cried and pleaded to go back home to Belgium. We loathed living in that house as it was situated accross from a funeral home which gave us children the creeps.

We all endured living in a one room unit for three long months. We had to make do with a shower stall instead of the bathtub we had been accustomed to. We washed our dishes in the tiny bathroom sink. Mother was on a strict budget of $20.00 per week as all other money went to pay the rent, bus fare, purchase father's cigarettes, and to repay the $500.00 loan from a friend. It was, without doubt, a very depressing and difficult time in which to get accustomed to this new Country.

Not surprisingly, my parents' marriage went downhill from there. My mother's headaches became worse. She noticed that people used a lot of perfume, strong after shave and unpleasant deodorants which triggered instant headaches. She could not for the life of her figure out why the general public in Canada used so much heavily scented products, but then again it was a different Country and a different culture. To this day, fragrances are still a problem for my mother. Even my sisters and I are sensitive to this malaise.

Living under these circumstances was a nightmare, but there we all were and there was no way to turn back the clock. Even after moving to a half-decent apartment, the problems kept escalating from bad to worse.

When mother had had enough she made the decision to file for divorce. She would rather face the challenge of being alone with her children, than living with father's constant mood swings, and, since he never did take a part in our up-bringing, she knew she would be better off without him.

I can't imagine how a father of eight would never once change a diaper, or help to bathe or feed his children. But my father lived life as if he were a swinging bachelor.

When the divorce was finalized in 1974, the Court ordered my father to pay to my mother $35.00 per week, which he did for the first six weeks. Thereafter, my mother did not get a cent from him. No wonder I sound bitter!

THE MAGIC GREEN PILL

As time went by, things slowly improved for us. Mother was much happier. The only obstacle remaining was her headaches. Who could blame her for those, considering all she had already lived through. She was obliged, against her better judgment, to rely on over-the-counter medication to control the now unbearable pain.

When the headaches became more frequent, mother noticed that the pain was not of the same pattern as before. It was perplexing and aggravating to figure out the appropriate pain killer for her headaches.

As no one doctor had been able to provide a so called "magic cure", my mother took it upon herself to do a little research by purchasing some books on the subject of headaches.

My mother learned that a headache was not just a headache. The enormous variety of headaches astonished her. The books referred to migraines, allergies, stress, atmospheric pressure (weather change), clusters and others. She began to understand the differences in headaches and their levels of intensity, but beyond self-testing instructions, no specific solutions were offered other than to avoid the cause of the headaches.

Avoiding the cause of her headaches was next to impossible. How do you tell your co-workers not to wear any perfume because you are allergic to odours? How can you control the weather if it is too cold, too hot or too humid? How do you figure out which foods you are allergic to? The process could take forever because you have to try one food for a few days before you can determine if you should eliminate it from your diet.

My mother relied on her nose. If she smelled something which ruffled her feathers, she kept away from it. She confirmed that her nose was right, when she accepted a few dinner invitations where it was impossible to decline the items on the menu.

On occasion she had attempted to explain her allergies, but found that her friends and relatives thought that it was just an excuse and an attempt to use her headaches to decline to eat or to drink wine or alcohol. So as not to offend anyone further, she decided to do the inviting herself. This way she could control the menu.

Those readers who have allergies can sympathize with the impossibility of avoiding certain triggering factors.

As aspirins no longer had any effect on my mother's headaches, she had to figure out the complexity of which over-the-counter medication was strong enough for her pain. She decided to take a chance and asked the pharmacist's opinion. The pharmacist sympathized with her because he too suffered from headaches. He gave her a single little green capsule at the cost of twenty-five cents. He confidently assured her not to worry and to go home and take the capsule and let him know how well it worked.

Mother took the capsule at five o'clock in the afternoon and went to lie down. She ended up sleeping until the next morning. When she woke up at her usual time of seven a.m., she could hardly believe she had slept the entire night. This was the first time in ages that she had been able to sleep for so long without waking up.

All of us children greeted her with a smile at breakfast. Giggling, we told her that we had tried to wake her up, but nothing worked. We had emptied the two liter ice cream bucket and watched television past our bedtime. Mother smiled and said that we had deserved the ice cream as we had to be our own cooks the previous evening. It crossed her mind that perhaps she had been given a strong sleeping pill, but such was not the case because she remained pain-free for an entire week before returning to the pharmacist with the good news.

He kindly told her she could purchase one capsule at a time as required. He knew that my mother would not abuse this medication and was happy to have been able to help her.

I must tell you that my mother never overslept again. That had been just one incident and understandable considering that the pain had vanished and relieved her to the point where she was able to get the rest she needed. Mother managed with one capsule every ten days or so, and kept this up for about one year.

One day she went to pick up her precious pill, but the pharmacist was not there. The replacement pharmacist advised her that the regular pharmacist had gone on holidays. Mother found it strange that the pharmacist had not told her in advance that he was going on holidays and had not provided her with a couple of extra pills to tide her over. She informed the new pharmacist of her condition, but he was unable to give her the capsule as he did not know its name. Unfortunately, my mother also did not know the name of the medication as the pharmacist had never disclosed the name of the pill.

Regrettably, the old pharmacist never returned. Mother was informed later that the pharmacy had been sold and that they could not provide her with the whereabouts of her pharmacist. She had no other choice but to explain the situation to the new pharmacist who could only suggest trying a 222. She had never taken a 222 before but soon discovered that it was no match for the magic green pill.

The pain was by now acute, and the only way she could moderately control it was to take two 222 pills every four hours. She objected to the quantity of the 222's required to relieve the pain.

Except for the nasty headaches, my mother was otherwise in good health. Over the years she had been complimented by many people and even by a few doctors who could hardly believe that she was the mother of eight children. That is how fit she looked then and still does.

PHYSIOTHERAPY AND CHIROPRACTIC ADJUSTMENT

Several times mother had sought advice and treatment from neurologists. They subjected her to all imaginable tests because they wished to be certain that the headaches were not associated with a potentially serious underlying illness. As she anxiously awaited the results, the doctors only confirmed what she already knew, that she had "multiple chronic headaches". What was of immence consolation was that there were never any tumors or other structural abnormalities detected.

The specialist ordered her to follow a couple of specific treatments that had been found to be helpful to some patients with a similar affliction. The treatment consisted of physiotherapy and chiropractic adjustments. The doctor thought that perhaps some neck manipulation would help, which in her case did not. Strong traction on her neck had no effect.

On the contrary, the last one was so bad that she literally came home in tears declaring that she would never go for such exaggerated treatment again.

To this day she remains skeptical about any neck disturbance that is supposed to help migraines. These manipulations of the neck, we believe, benefit only a limited number of patients.

The application of hot and cold packs were also ineffective on my mother. They only gave her an additional sinus headache. So much for these experiments. The outcome of all this experimentation was more headaches and several different prescriptions to try out over the next few months. No change was observed exept that the medication upset her stomach and made her sleepy.

My mother began to resent going to the doctor because it seemed to lead nowhere. Once again she was at point zero, and had no choice but to continue taking the 222's.

On a couple of occasions she was gripped by such intolerable pain that we had to take her to emergency in the hope that she would be given a "real" pain killer. After several hours of waiting, she was told that people with headaches should not come to Emergency and waste the physicians' time. Nothing was given to her, not even a dose of sympathy. She was astonished at the reception she received from a medical practitioner, but the worst was yet to come.

Mother was left with many unanswered questions. How was it possible that living in this day and age with a health care system which spends billlions of dollars in research and state of the art technology, which produces a great number of doctors and specialists, could give her no answers?

Disillusioned more than ever, mother decided to forego the services of the medical profession.

Something that my mother learned much later, but was not aware of at the time, was that all medicines, whether prescribed or over-the-counter, have side effects. This is a serious and critical factor that all consumers should be aware of and should use extreme caution about. People still think that if you get it at the pharmacy, it is harmless. Don't be fooled! Any substance taken for a prolonged period of time will eventually harm you. Please avoid this at all costs and especially do not mix medication. To prevent toxic liver damage from medication, ask your doctor for periodic blood tests to monitor any irregularities.

I CHOOSE A CAREER

As these events were occurring, all of us children were growing up and trying to make career choices. From early on I had always had an interest in the medical field. Being uncertain which direction I should pursue, and unwilling to incur high tuition fees in medical school, I, at the age of twenty, determined to find employment in one of the city hospitals to get an inside look to guide my future choice.

The summer of 1977, being vacation time for many people, I got lucky and was hired as a nurses' aid. I was chosen to work on the rotating team, which meant that I reported every morning to the head nurse to be assigned to whichever department was short-handed. I truly enjoyed my work. My curiosity knew no bounds and I learned much.

I must admit that I worked fast and was extremely efficient at my job. My secret was to arrive fifteen minutes before my shift and skipping the morning break, which for me was unnecessary, as I had one hour for lunch and another half-hour break in the afternoon. For me, being ahead in my work made all the difference to my day and I felt good going home knowing that all my duties had been taken care of.

I worked as a nurse's aid for one year and gained valuable experience. Unfortunately, none of the research I did at the time brought me any closer to discovering the solution to my mother's headaches. As the doctors were stumped, the next move was up to us. And move we did!

WE MOVE TO BRITISH COLUMBIA

My mother and I decided to make British Columbia our destination. We hoped that the mild weather would be in mother's favour. It did not take long to find out that the four seasons in British Columbia were very much alike.

If anything, the long periods of rain seemed to make mother's headaches worse.

We also discovered that the medical system in British Columbia differed in a number of respects from the system back East. In B.C., before going to a specialist, one was required to have a family physician who would make a referral to a specialist.

Although we did not approve of this system, we had little choice. We still believe it is in the best interests of the patient to have direct access to a specialist who could deal with the patient's concerns in a more timely fashion.

The provincial government is of the opinion that going through a family doctor saves money. This raises the question: is the alleged saving worth the life and health of the patient? Certainly a balanced budget is desirable and cuts are needed, but not at the expense of our lives.

If a patient must make numerous visits to his family doctor before being referred to a specialist, where is the saving? Who considers what the patient endures when his health deteriorates while he wastes valuable time in visit after visit to the family doctor, and spends money on prescription after prescription.

It is said that if you have a problem, go directly to the source. So why make costly detours? Admittedly, the right answers are sometimes hard to find and a family doctor should not risk the health of his patient in pretending to know better than a specialist.

Maybe it is time for the Medical Association to re-assess its values and its contribution to society. While everyone wants equal access to common resources, some inevitably take more than their fair share.

I believe that governmental control is largely responsible for the decay in our society. Governments are hungry for power and when expenses exceed their budgets, they pass the problem on to "the little people" as we are often referred to. Taxing the public to death is not the answer! We all have to budget for our living expenses and free spending becomes difficult when half our earned income goes towards the national debt and other unnecessary governmental expenses.

Our government says that our medical system is expensive and levies higher taxes. But what does it cost us when we go for a visit to the doctor:

- time from work without pay;
- cost of taxi fare;
- cost of parking if you drive there;
- risk of losing your job if you must make numerous visits, schedule blood tests, x rays, therapy, surgery;
- baby-sitting expenses;
- lengthy delays in the waiting room due to overbooking patients.

No wonder some people aggravate their condition by postponing as long as possible a visit to the doctor in an attempt to avoid these stressful circumstances.

As we approach the year 2000, we wonder if we have progressed at all. We have more doctors than ever, yet we have more patients with diseases than ever before. People are becoming increasingly unhappy with their medical services.

The quality of care is diluting and becoming progressively worse. In due course, if nothing is done, people will stay sicker longer and will not be able to return to work as originally anticipated. The repercussions are staggering.

Matters can still be changed, but our broken down system will take years to fix. Every illness relies on the art of healing and calls for tranquility without tranquilizers. We must all contribute our fair share for we have nothing to lose and everything to gain.

CHAPTER III

The Nightmares Begin

MOTHER CONSULTS A GENERAL PRACTIONER

Mother was nowhere close to finding peace. She could not perceive how a general practitioner could help her when all attempts of the specialists had failed. None could provide her with answers, only empty promises that someday medicine might advance to the point of providing her with a solution.

Empty promises were of no consolation to my mother who, facing a new breed of so called family practitioner, had to explain her condition all over again. This particular family physician seemed rather pleasant, but his attention lacked enthusiasm. Within minutes she was sent on her way with a prescription of Cafergot and a referral to a neurologist. Mother was somewhat displeased with this hasty treatment but did in due course consult the neurologist.

She later found out from another doctor, that the neurologist had written a confidential report that mother was in perfect health and that her headaches were in all likelihood imaginary. This discovery left my mother feeling numb and angry. Needless to say, her optimism started to dwindle in the face of one frustrating roadblock after another.

This was just the first of many such remarks my mother was to hear about her headaches and the other complications which followed. It marked the beginning of the growing mistrust and resentment she was to feel towards the medical profession in general.

We are brought up to respect the skills and knowledge of doctors, a respect which cannot be sustained in the face of the gradual decline of the medical profession.

MASSAGE THERAPY AS AN ALTERNATIVE

These are not simple times we live in and one cannot but express frustration over the attitudes of our physicians. While the future holds promise, present reality needs serious modification because it is hurting patient services. Note the increasing waiting lists for surgery.

Diseases can be largely avoidable if adequate preventive measures are taken. We also know that no one person has all the right answers, so every person who does have knowledge should make it his business, for the benefit of others, to pass it on.

That is something which I have been attempting to do ever since having established my own private and independent massage therapy service.

During the year I worked as a nurse's aid and witnessed on a daily basis the constant pain and suffering patients endure, I had chosen to become a masseuse. I thought that the only way that anyone could put a stop to human pain is through prevention, so the idea of working in the preventive field strongly appealed to me.

Prevention is extremely effective and is a pain-free treatment. Massage requires the study of anatomy, physiology and the use of skilled hands and brain for its healing result. Its purpose is to produce a therapeutic effect on the tissues of the nervous, muscular and respiratory systems of the body. It also serves to stimulate blood supply and foster confidence. That is something a machine cannot do.

Massage is now becoming more accepted as an effective means of relieving emotional and physical stress, relaxing and simply feeling good. Contrary to common belief, massage therapy is not only prescribed for or administered to the sick and injured, and is not the exclusive indulgence of the rich and famous.

It was developed for use on muscles and the whole human structure and as such is beneficial to all individuals. It provides comfort and healing to countless sufferers, relieves tension, stiffness, spasms, and by relaxing tight and aching muscles, soothes away certain headaches. It increases flexibility, encourages muscles to work at full capacity, and induces a general sense of well-being. A good friction massage adds a healthy glow to your complexion by boosting blood circulation.

The daily monotony of our occupations tends to restrict muscle activity resulting in muscular soreness. A massage which includes ruffling the muscles in all directions with stretches, pulls, applied pressure and other movements, provides a burst of energy. It relieves psychological stress and can improve a person's state of mind.

As far as frequency of massage is concerned, I would say that the more often you have it, the greater its benefits. I would suggest that once a week is ideal, but even once a month can be of benefit.

The environment in which you receive massage is very important. It must be clean, warm, quiet, with no distractions or interruptions. Low volume background music adds to the soothing effect. The therapist must be well mannered and courteous. He or she should have clean nails, and soft yet firm hands. A professionally trained therapist is one who makes people feel at ease, has patience, and shows interest in the client's well being.

Over the years in which I have been treating people, I have seen a great increase in the use of massage as a successful and drug-free alternative to combatting stress. I am very happy to report clients that were able through massage to completely eliminate their need for tranquilizers, muscle relaxants and sleeping aids.

Massage is essential to your good health and should be part of your life! I have always regarded it as an art form. Just as a sculptor magically transforms a block of clay into a beautiful masterpiece, I let my hands flow uninterruptedly through their motion to the sound of peaceful music to rid the body of all distress.

Even skeptics have had to admit that such varied forms of art as dancing, painting, sculpting, playing and listening to music, and yes, massage, can reach parts of the human body that conventional treatments cannot. A massage treatment, varying in duration from as little as a half hour, to a maximum of one and a half hours, provides the patient with ample time to expose his buried emotions.

As a therapist, I of course, get to hear a great deal of people's complaints. Over time, clients develop a sense of security and feel comfortable enough to confide their personal problems to me. Regardless of what they actually express, clients, more than anything, just want to be heard. So I listen.

Eight out of ten clients consistently complain of medical problems and the lack of time and attention they receive from their doctors. Quite often, their doctors can do little for them so time and again they return to me for massage therapy.

Since becoming established in 1983, I have had the opportunity to treat many people. One of the most common complaints they come to me for is an aching back. That is a pain that their general practitioners do not feel comfortable with so they prescribe Tylenol and send them home to bed. Eventually, family doctors will make referrals to chiropractors or a physiotherapists.

It is not my intention to criticize any of these recommended treatments, which if applied with great care, benefit millions of people. Massage therapy is usually last on the list of recommended treatments, so we massage therapists get an earful from dissatisfied clients. I will therefore share the concern of some of my clients who wish to remain anonymous and believe that their complaints won't make a difference.

What they object to the most is the duration of treatments they receive from physiotherapists and chiropractors. The Physios are known to employ the same routine, which is to handle three or four patients at one time. While one waits for the hot or cold pack to take effect, another is in traction (sustained therapeutic pulling on a limb), and yet another receives ultrasonic waves (used for various joint and muscle disorders).

As for the chiropractors, most everyone says the same thing, "Crick-crack, two minutes and you're out the door". This is no way to treat people! I have to question their methods as healing requires gentleness and most of all, time. Rushing people through treatment every few minutes is not going to fix their problems any time soon.

The objective and primary responsibility of a healer, whether conventional or otherwise, is to use his knowledge to the best of his ability to ensure a successful recovery for his patient. More often than not, disorders linger because of the lack of time allotted to a patient's recovery. The physician's general preference is to take the quick and easy approach and treat the symptom rather than look for the cause. Hence he prescribes tranquilizers to a patient suffering from tension, rather than recommending massage therapy to reduce the emotional and physical stress that may be causing the tension.

Remember that anything purporting to be a "quick fix" is not the answer. I wish that the general populace could disabuse itself of the notion that its state of health depends primarily on medical intervention. To this day I am angry at a system which permits unlimited consultations with doctors which are certainly more costly to the taxpayer than regular visits with a massage therapist.

Week after week I hear people say "I saw my doctor several times and my back still hurts". Or, "I've used up my twelve visits with the chiropractor and my twelve sessions of physio and still I do not feel much improved". Doctors cannot be expected to spend the same amount of time with a patient that a massage therapist does. My success is largely due to the fact that I invest an adequate amount of time in treating my clients. The average ten minute visit with the doctor does not allow time to delve into the patient's history, to review applicable medical literature and to determine the best course of treatment for that particular patient's problem.

For many, massage therapy is a last recourse because the medical system continues to operate under the delusion that massage is a leisure activity. A service that relaxes you and makes you feel good cannot possibly be as beneficial as other services. Baloney!

It would certainly make more sense if all available treatment options were presented to a patient prior to beginning any one treatment. Instead, doctors send their patients back and forth from one place to the next. After weeks and months of this merry-go-round, it is no wonder that a patient's inflammatory condition has become more aggravated.

Health care is for all, not just for a particular type of person, and as such must address not only physical symptoms but social problems as well.

For most people, eliminating stiffness, stress, sore joints, etc. will take two or three sessions of massage. If the condition is chronic, then regular treatments are advisable. When massage therapy achieves positive results, it should be maintained for preventive reasons.

It annoys me considerably when I see a person limping into my office with his back bent awkwardly and grimacing in pain. Such was the case for one of my clients. He told me that his doctor had diagnosed him with Sciatica about three months before. He was given no medication nor was any other course of treatment suggested. He was simply told that it would take six months to get better and that he would just have to wait it out.

Sciatica is a condition of severe pain in the lower back which runs down the back of the thigh and leg. It is caused by direct pressure on a nerve. In some cases it is associated with degeneration of an intervertebral disk (fiberlike tissue found between spinal vertebrae). Why would a doctor want to leave his patient in such pain?

I do not know of a case where Sciatica dissipated on its own. I suffer from Sciatica myself on occasion and the only thing that helps is the "side to side, hold, stretch". It is essential to do this routine which is almost always effective. It has not failed me or my clients.

I make my clients practice the stretching routine in my office and give them proper and simple instructions on how to do it at home. A massage treatment prior to the stretch helps to limber up, but the stretch itself must be done a couple times a day in order to alleviate the problem.

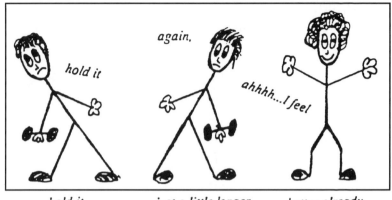

hold it | just a little longer | better already.

In order for the side stretch to be effective, you must first stand up straight, with feet slightly apart, and holding a wrist weight or hand weight of two or three pounds, lean towards the side of the body in which you hold the weight. Retain this position for at least three minutes, then do the other side. Yes, I know it is painful, but it works by helping to unlock the compression on the nerve.

PATIENTS' RIGHTS

My advice to people is "Don't say it doesn't work until you've tried it, and do not forget that your health comes first". You alone control what you want and what you do not want. It is your body and your own decision! Don't use stress as an excuse, you must take the initial step towards whatever you wish to accomplish. Simply remember that a healthy life is a richer and happier one.

Being healthy does not mean taking things for granted. We are the ones responsible for evaluating each and every course of treatment that may be recommended to us. Just because certain doctors have a tendency to be single-minded in their opinions and our ideas don't carry much weight with them, who other than ourselves know best what is going on inside of us. We expect doctors to have the ability to make us feel at ease, to show an interest and get us to talk about ourselves. Instead, they try to intimidate those of us who come in with too many questions, because answering them is not their favourite subject or their strong point.

If a doctor remains evasive, just remember that as a patient you have rights, more than you can know, so be strong, fight back and most of all, do what feels right for you! Use common sense. Don't leave home without it.

From the Health Naturally magazine June/July 1993:

KNOW YOUR PATIENTS' RIGHTS

In a large, impersonal health care system it is easy to forget that you have certain rights. you are the customer and you are in charge. Those who perform health services for you have an obligation both to respect your rights and to meet your standards of performance. Know your rights. Insisting on them could save your life.

1. **You Have the Right to Complete Information**

   You have the right to receive complete information and to have an explanation of your condition, treatment and chances (if any) of recovery – in layman's terms. You also have the right to an interpreter, if needed.

   You have the right to know the nature and purpose of procedures, the hazards and possible side effects they may cause, and by whom they may be done – whether by qualified practitioner or by medical student.

   You have the right to expect that your doctor will summon a more capable colleague when diagnosis or treatment is beyond his capabilities.

You have the right to know, by name, the physician responsible for your care.

You have the right to a full explanation of your bill.

2. You Have the Right to Refuse Consent

You must be given enough information regarding proposed procedures and their alternatives – in order to give informed consent before treatment. You then have the right to consent or to refuse such treatments – as well as to know what other treatments there are to choose from. Some doctors may be reluctant to tell you about alternate methods of healing.

You have a right to obtain a second opinion from another medical doctor, or from other healers who use entirely different principles.

Beware of "all inclusive" consent forms. Do not hesitate to refuse to sign consent forms or to modify them by crossing out parts. Your consent is valid only if it is voluntary and informed.

3. You Have the Right to Privacy

No matter what your economic status is, or what source of payment you use, you have the right to keep your records private and confidential. Your records and any information about your case can only be released to another person with your consent. The records themselves, in most cases, are the property of the doctor and the hospital, but the information contained in them is yours.

[Note: Access to your records, however, is available to researchers, the courts (through subpoena), and public health officials (for notifiably communicable diseases).]

You have the right to know the information contained in your records and the right to keep this information confidential.

You can obtain a copy of your records by giving written authorization to a sympathetic doctor, who can then send your authorization to the institution that has your records. They will send your records to this doctor and s/he will give them to you.

4. You Have the Right to Refuse to be in Experiments

You have the right to know whether you are being used in teaching, research or experimentation – and the right to refuse to participate.

5. You Have the Right to be Treated in Emergencies

You have the right to be treated in an emergency by a hospital and by a doctor – unless that doctor can be assured that treatment can and will be given by others.

6. You Have the Right to Leave

You have the right to leave the hospital or doctor's office whenever you decide to and even when advised against it. You may be asked to sign a form releasing responsibility for any harm that might come to you.

[Note: except if you have been involuntarily committed to a mental institution.]

7. You Have the Right to Quality Care

You have the right to considerate, respectful, suitable, good quality, humane care. You also have the right to courtesy, respect, dignity and continuity of care.

8. You Have the Right to Switch

You have the right to choose your doctor(s) and to change doctor at any time. Shopping for a doctor is no different from shopping for any service. Once you choose, there is nothing obligating you to continue as patient. It is advantageous, however, to find a doctor with whom you can develop a good rapport – and to stay with him or her so that you will have continuity of care.

These rights are mentioned by the Canadian Medical Association in its Code of Ethics, the World Medical Association in its International Code of Medical Ethics, and the Canadian Council on Hospital Accreditation in the preamble of its guide to hospital accreditation. You can obtain copies from these organizations or from a public library.

Source: The above list of rights was first published in PATIENTS' RIGHTS HANDBOOK, by Jerry Green, MD and Tom McLaughlin in the late 1970s. Since that time, our health care system has grown even larger and less personal. Thus, our need to be aware of our rights as patients is more timely now than ever.

(end of article)

A two way exchange between the professional and the patient would ensure continued growth and development of healing therapies. All of us must at some point in our lives sweep aside failures because ahead of us there are success stories that we can build on. Today's science is continously trying to cure something, but it will not cure it all, at least no time soon. The point has come when more effort must be invested in prevention rather than in trying to cure the incurable.

Life is actually very simple and it is up to us to add life to our years and years to our life. Sometimes it is hard to attain our objective and even harder to maintain it, but learning is a part of life and, in the end, what is most important is what works for us. It is a question of our attitudes and how we wish to deal with life. Mistakes don't have to be repeated as long as we have access to available information to allow us to make the right decisions for ourselves.

Don't plan a treatment only to quit it a few days later. If you do, you'll only hurt yourself more. In all likelihood, you have already endured many medical inefficiencies, lived through long and stressful periods of waiting and hoping that the medical verdict will not be too bad, before deciding to take matters into your own hands and become involved in your own treatment.

A good place to start doing your own research is your local library. Better yet, some medical schools and teaching hospitals have their own libraries which are open to the public. Don't be shy, ask the librarian for help. The librarian will direct you to reference books and indexes appropriate to your particular subject. Start reading and take notes on the condition or ailment you are stricken with, and photocopy any pertinent articles. Be prepared to spend a lot of hours reading. You may be overwhelmed by the complexity of medical texts because they are often difficult, if not impossible, to figure out. But have faith in the power of your mind.

Goodness comes from the heart,

Just as intelligence comes from the spirit.

GARLIC/COGNAC RECIPE FOR RHEUMATISM

I came accross this recipe in a magazine. I've been drinking this concoction for the past two years, and I can honestly say that my hands (because of my work as a therapist) would be crippled in pain without it.

Garlic has been credited with many properties but few are aware of its benefits for rheumatism.

To alleviate pain, skin the cloves of four large heads of garlic and marinate them in 450ml of French brandy for about ten days.

Take half a teaspoon of the marinade diluted in half a glass of water (room temperature) first thing every morning. Do not put the potion in the refrigerator.

When preparing the magic potion, use a glass bottle or jar and cover the top with foil paper to keep the garlic odour from evaporating (it smells terrible but it's worth it to be pain free).

This recipe is for a lifetime and is truly meant to be passed on.

Rheumatism: any of a variety of disorders marked by inflammation, degeneration, or metabolic derangement of the connective tissue structure, especially the joints and related structures, and attended by pain, stiffness, or limitation of motion.

MOTHER SUFFERS ANOTHER SETBACK

My mother, who had by now faced endless medical disappointments, always told us to be prepared for the worst, so that when it came, it would not seem so terrible.

In December of 1989, at the age of fifty-seven, mother had gained only a few extra pounds during her menopause years, fluctuating between 125 and 130 pounds. As fate would have it, she was suddenly stricken with pain on the right side of the abdominal area, accompanied with bloating and digestive problems.

She went to her family doctor, her second since coming to British Columbia. The doctor insisted that her malaise was nothing to worry about and was all part of aging. My mother did not buy this diagnosis. She insisted on tests, and the doctor, despite his opinion that tests were not necessary, finally complied.

One week later, the doctor had to admit my mother had been right. Her x-ray showed several calcified densities in the right upper quadrant, which could represent gallstones within the gall bladder. The doctor told mother that clinical correlation was recommended in such a case, but that he felt that the procedure was not necessary at this time, citing that many people lived with their gallstones without any complications.

Mother did not argue with the doctor. She knew how she felt and that somehow she would get her surgery. She asked the doctor for a referral to a specialist for a second opinion (a patient's right). To mother's disbelief, the doctor flatly refused her request. The doctor's attitude did not seem right, it "smelled fishy".

Until we could find another solution, we decided to read up on gall bladder problems to give us an idea of how to proceed.

As time went by, my mother became progressively worse. Her weight continued to rise and her abdominal area was extensively bloated and painful. As she was still suffering from her continous headaches, she went back to her doctor for a prescription of Cafergot, which relieves migraine headaches and other headaches caused by dilated blood vessels. Mother was also taking Percocet, a narcotic which blocks pain messages to the brain and spinal cord. For her, only the combination of the two taken together worked on her headaches.

On that visit, the doctor was still unwilling to send her to a specialist. Instead he sent her home with a prescription for 200 of each of the pills. She couldn't believe it, for this was clearly saying to her: "Don't bother me for a while". At this point, she felt that the time had come to find another family doctor, as she was no longer willing to be mistreated by this one.

MOTHER SEES A SPECIALIST IN INTERNAL MEDICINE

Some weeks went by before we were able to find a specialist in internal medicine to assess mother's gall bladder problem. She had to wait six weeks for an appointment, and since it was a non-referred visit, we had to pay a sixty dollar fee. We did not object to this. After all, life is worth more than a few dollars!

When she saw the specialist, he performed an immediate ultrasound and confirmed that surgery had to be performed as soon as possible. Her condition had become severe and the operation was to take place within a few weeks. It would have been done sooner except that there was a hospital strike at the time and each surgeon was limited to one or two operations per week.

Mother had the surgery in May of 1990 and recuperated very well. She was pleased to soon lose those extra pounds. She was now very cautious with her diet as she no longer had a gall bladder.

GET TO KNOW YOUR BODY

You do not need a gall bladder to live, but as you are born with it, it must serve some purpose. You should know that the liver, gall bladder and pancreas, together with the digestive tract, make up the digestive system.

The liver has many functions; one of which is to make bile (a green fluid that passes into the duodenum, the first part of the small intestine immediately below the stomach). To help break down fats bile is stored in the gall bladder which is connected to the duodenum via the bile duct (a tube-like channel for carrying fluids or other materials from one organ to another).

The pancreas is located beneath the stomach and produces juices that pass along the pancreatic duct, into the duodenum where they help break down carbohydrates, proteins and fats.

Carbohydrates can be either starches or sugars. They are the chief energy sources of the body. We consume them in the form of cereals, flour products, fruits and vegetables.

Proteins are found in meats, fish, eggs and cheese. There are also a variety of vegetable proteins which are found in beans, peas and other legumes. Proteins are also present in grains and therefore in breads.

Fats are found in plant foods such as olives and peanuts, and in meats. Fat provides energy. Excess fats are laid down in the body in the form of fatty tissue. Even though it may provide some benefits as insulation, this fat can cause serious health problems.

Remember, your food is your fuel and if you neglect your engine, as we might call it, it won't remain running for long.

The first piece of advice is that you must consult a doctor from the very beginning, regardless of how insignificant your symptom may be. If your doctor tells you there is nothing wrong with you and you feel otherwise (as my mother did), insist on blood tests, x-rays or ultrasounds, if necessary.

It is the doctor's duty and your right to find out what is causing your ill health. No matter what, do not give up until you get to the bottom of things.

One very important thing to do, is to always ask for a copy of your lab test results. This way you can follow the ups and downs of your progress, and at the same time become a full and participating contributor to your own treatment.

Don't worry and do not panic if you are unable to understand the readings on the lab reports because with your results comes a reference range you can look at to see where you stand. If the test numbers you see read above or below a given normal range, then you can start asking questions such as "What brought this on?". Ask for the known causes and available remedies.

If you know what is best for you, don't wait for the problem to escalate. If you hope that whatever ailment you have will simply disappear, you're wasting your precious time. The longer you wait to be attended to, the longer it will take you to heal, and in the worst cast scenario not heal at all. If this is not enough encouragement, then think of the anguish you and those around you will suffer. Remember that if you don't become involved, you'll become a subject of modern science. Always be prepared for highs and lows and expect to get a different opinion from each doctor you consult. Their recommendations have come to be as capricious as the fluctuations of the stock market.

All of us are different hence our physiological needs differ. Whatever treatment cures one, or millions of others, may not cure you! I say this again not just because of mother's gall bladder experience, but because of what followed.

MOTHER GOES TO A NEW FAMILY DOCTOR

For all those that have been, are, or will be caught in similar horrors, we wish to share with you the information and experience we acquired through my mother's entire ordeal. Only people who have suffered comparably can appreciate what she went through. Neglect of that kind should not be allowed to exist.

In our adversities, we never gave up or lost hope. Mother always had this incredible strength to endure miseries, but her condition became so bad that she herself had forgotten what feeling good and healthy felt like.

70

Despite the multiple complications that were continuously arising, mother's doctor remained quite evasive and certainly managed to keep her off track by repeatedly telling her that she was okay, that her weight gain was part of aging, and that the severity of her long-standing and irremediable headaches was due to a decreased pain tolerance in older people.

Mother found it insulting and unacceptable to be told, without investigation or analysis of other factors, that women problems are most often caused by old age or menopause. Unimpressed, mother did not accept her physician's theory, especially when she delicately implied that she was most certainly on a very rich calorie diet, which was not true. She urged her to start a regimen consisting of soup only, morning, lunch and dinner, accompanied with a slice of rye bread. She also recommended that she join the Y.W.C.A. for swimming and beginner's aerobics classes.

On that note, mother left having agreed to try the soup diet, but in no way was she going to follow the exercise program, for the reason that her daily one-hour walk was becoming increasingly exhausting due to breathing difficulties, general physical weakness and ankle soreness. Some time later we discovered that her symptoms had been labelled as "due to overuse symptoms and perhaps improper shoes". This was an incorrect assessment, and just one example of the many misguided communications among mother's doctors. We truly began to wonder if there was any significance to the description of doctors as <u>practicing</u> physicians!

In any case, while mother had nothing against following doctor's orders, she knew perfectly well, better than anyone else, how she felt and what she was and was not capable of. She knew that waking up with pain, living in pain, and going to bed in pain was not normal. It had become physically and mentally exhausting. At this point mother could only wonder "What's next?"

MOTHER'S MISHAP AT THE DENTIST'S

What came next occurred after a routine check-up at the dentist's office. Being the first person to arrive at the dentist's office, she immediately picked-up on his very noticeable fresh-smelling aftershave lotion. She knew it would set off a headache, but what she did not expect was the outbreak of blisters in her mouth several hours after being examined without latex gloves.

This was a blatant case of negligence on the dentist's part. Medical practitioners take strict precautions to avoid contracting bacteria or infections from patients, but who protects patients from their neglect? For mother, that day was spoiled and she went without lunch and dinner because of the irritation in her mouth.

This incident parallels a similar occurrence several years prior, when mother had kissed her companion who had just refreshed his breath with mouth wash. He had given her "the kiss of death". Needless to say he was later asked to refrain from using it if he wanted to kiss mother again.

THE IMITREX SCARE

Time after time, mother would react to some seemingly harmless substance. We heard about a new breakthrough medication called "Imitrex", apprently tailormade for migraine sufferers. For a brief moment, mother allowed herself to hope that maybe this would finally be a solution to her miseries. Her doctor, however, told her that the drug was absolutely not for her because it was specifically for migraines.

Mother continued to use her regular medication for several months before returning to the doctor to renew her prescription. Upon entering the doctor's consultation room, she noticed that the doctor was acting rather strangely. Without much explanation the doctor told mother that it was imperative that she come off her customary medication and immediately start on Imitrex (Sumatriptan Succinate 100).

Mother was puzzled as to why the doctor should so suddenly change her mind and asked some questions about the new drug. She enquired as to the physical reaction she could expect upon taking the Imitrex without gradually being taken off her regular prescription. It is no secret that you cannot quit one drug cold turkey and switch to another without some kind of adverse reaction. But the doctor told her she had no choice, as her recent blood test indicated a mild case of Hepatitis C (inflammation of the liver).

The effects of Hepatitis C manifest themselves in jaundice, cirrhosis of the liver, loss of muscle strength and easy bruising or bleeding. At its worst, Hepatitis C leads a sufferer to fall into a coma or develop liver cancer.

The doctor advised that she need not be alarmed and that by switching medication, the hepatitis would disappear in due time.

Mother thought the doctor was acting in an unusually hasty and insistent manner totally out of character for her. The doctor told her to go off the Cafergot and Percocet for a period of 48 hours and then start taking the Imitrex. Mother asked if she could wait at least until after the Easter long week-end before going off her regular prescription. She knew she could not go six hours without pain medication, let alone 48 hours. She felt the transition might require close supervision and that the Easter holiday was definitely not the best time to switch medication.

The doctor replied that mother should do her best to force herself not to take any medication for at least 24 hours. The doctor added that if worse came to worse, mother could go to Emergency. That was no consolation as mother knew from previous experience that the the staff at Emergency could only act if the family physician was out of town and had left written instructions.

Upon leaving the doctor's office, my mother and I tried to analize the doctor's orders. We found it questionable that a person diagnosed with hepatitis C virus and one who was for years dependant on pain killers, would be left unsupervised to attempt on her own the delicate task of withdrawing from prescription medication. Surely such a person should be admitted into a care facility and kept under the watchful eye of trained staff. Bitterly, we felt that the new generation of physician was a far cry from Marcus Welby.

Personally, I feel we live in a culture of neglect. Young people are entering college at an age where they have not yet learned personal commitment, having formed only minimal authentic attachments to others. Medical school does not teach the ethics of concern. Medicine has escalated into a major industry lacking in responsibility and accountability. It seems that a physician's primary concern is not the quality of care for the patient, but how much he is going to get paid.

Mother's circumstances illustrate perfectly well how powerless patients stand before the arrogance of science.

Imitrex, although market approved, was only in its early stages of use on the public, which to us meant that it had been "accepted for public experimentation". With no protection against a new substance, mother was reduced to a guinea pig.

While finding another general practitioner was again desirable, the few good ones can only be found by word of mouth. They are as difficult to find as a needle in a haystack.

As mother was left with no other option, she went to the pharmacist to fill her prescription for Imitrex. The pharmacist was uneasy about filling the prescription as her professional instinct agreed with mother's. She could only sympathize with mother and wish her good luck.

Mother headed home to face the next 24 hours. She developed a headache of unexpressable magnitude and spent a sleepless night. Good Friday approached but there was nothing "good" about it.

When mother took her first Imitrex pill, nothing happened. She waited as long as she could and four hours later took another one. As the drug kicked-in, mother began to feel strange and her head seemed as if it was about to blow off at any minute. It was a massive high blood-pressure headache.

Knowing that my mother needed urgent medical attention, I called the doctor's office first. I got a recorded message that the doctor was on call and could be reached on her pager. I tried her pager and left a message. We waited impatiently, and after thirty minutes I called again and left another message. Again we waited, and again I left two more messages.

A couple of hours went by and by now mother was in sheer agony. I tried a few massage techniques on my mother which have helped her in the past, but to no avail.

I took a chance and called a neurologist. To my surprise, a male voice answered. I asked to speak to Dr. _____. The telephone conversation went as follows:

Me: I'm calling in regards to what to do with my mother's reaction to Imitrex. (Description)

Dr.: Excuse me Miss (harsh tone of voice) but do you know what time this is?

Me: Yes Doctor, it's 8:30 in the morning.

Dr.: Don't you think it's a bit early to disturb me for someone who is not even my patient.

Me: But Doctor, since you're answering your own office number, I assume you aren't sleeping, and must be there for a reason. Please, can you at least advise me on what to do, after all, you're the specialist, or is that a mistake?

Dr.: I don't have time for this, go where everyone else goes, the Emergency.

Me: What if they don't know what to do?

Dr.: They'll think of something.

Me: (Thinking quickly) Could you at least tell me if it's safe for mother to go back on her Cafergot and Percocet without setting off another reaction?

Dr.: As I said Miss, your mother is not my patient, therefore you'll have to go through the normal procedures, see your G.P., get a referral and make an appointment with my secretary.

Me: My mother can't wait that long, she needs help today.

Dr.: Sorry! (Hanging up).

I called a taxi and together my mother and I headed for the hospital Emergency. There again we had to go through their so called normal procedures, which meant waiting several more hours before being attended to.

When mother's turn came, all they did was give her an anti-nausea injection, make her wait twenty minutes and tell her to go home and see her doctor on Tuesday. They told us that they had tried contacting mother's doctor for instructions, but had got no response either.

By that time I was more than a little frustrated. I apologized for my anger and insisted that they give me a prescription for 3 Cafergots and 3 Percocets to hold mother until Tuesday morning. All I got was a firm "No". They said "We're sorry, but at times we can't prescribe something without the patient's doctor's consent". I replied "It's rather strange that a doctor cannot prescribe without another's approval first. This is outrageous. Why are you a doctor anyway!" The doctor then said, "Sorry Miss. That's just the way it is", and disappeared. So again we called a taxi and headed home.

For mother, except for the absence of nausea, nothing had changed. By mid-afteroon I decided to call my sister to come over to watch our mother while I went out to hunt for her medication.

My first thought was to go to another hospital Emergency, explain the situation and beg for some medication. Upon further reflection I discarded that idea as I figured that they would most likely follow the same regulations and would not give out any medication without the doctor's approval. I opted to go to the pharmacy, not our usual one downtown as it would take too long to get there, but the one uptown which we went to on occasion. I was off in a flash.

I calmly approached the pharmacist who recognized me and asked how she could help. I simply said that my mother had run out of her medication sooner than expected, and if it was at all possible, could I get 3 Cafergots and 3 Percocets to tide her over until Tuesday. The pharmacist replied "No problem". I was overjoyed and even took a few extra seconds to call my sister from a pay phone so she could tell mother I was on my way home with the pills.

Oh yes, I must not forget to tell you that the pharmacist didn't even charge me for the pills, and, assuming that mother was too sick, offered to call the doctor herself on Tuesday to okay and fill out the rest of the regular prescription. I told her that it wouldn't be necessary because mother had to go see the doctor anyway. I felt a little guilty for not having told her the true story, but I felt that I had no choice.

When I got home, my mother and sister couldn't believe that I had actually pulled it off. But before rejoicing any further we had to wait and see if the pills would have their usual effect on mother's pain. After the catastrophic result with the Imitrex, we did not know what would happen next but felt it was a risk we had to take.

It took about a half hour before we saw any improvement. After another hour mother was almost back to her normal self. She slept that night and woke up to a happy Easter Sunday morning.

After the long weekend, mother returned to the doctor. She took a quick glance at mother and said, "Gee, you're looking well. I guess you're here for a repeat prescription of Imitrex". Mother replied in a severe tone, "Had you answered your beeper you would have found out that things didn't go well at all, and you're welcome to call the hospital Emergency for the details". Keeping her cool, the doctor reached into her pocket and pulled out her beeper. Checking the beeper, she said, "Oh my gosh, the battery is out". Mother could not believe that feeble excuse. One would assume that a doctor on call would think of verifying her pager, and would double check it if no calls had come in after one day, let alone after three days. All I can say is that the doctor simply did not care.

After a brief moment of reflection, the doctor looked at my mother and said, "Oh well, I guess I'll just put you back on your regular stuff" and proceeded to schedule her for a liver ultrasound and more blood tests. My mother said, "Fine!". She was worried that this latest incident had taken a toll on her physically, in the sense of energy loss, and the need for more medication to attenuate not only the headaches but also the additional physical pain which was probably caused by volume augmentation around the abdominal area. Mother wished that all this was due to old age, but her instinct said otherwise.

CHAPTER IV

Fatty Liver

MOTHER HAS AN ULTRASOUND

During the ultrasound my mother felt a considerable amount of pain. While performing the examination, the radiologist and an assisting doctor had spoken no words, but their exchange of eye contact had spoken volumes. Several other doctors had been called in to observe the screen showing direct images of her abdominal cavity. Mother asked the doctors what was going on, but they casually replied that she would have to wait and get the answer from her G.P.

So even before knowing the outcome of the ultrasound my mother expected a negative result of some kind. All we could do was sweat it out until the ultrasound results came in.

ULTRASOUND DIVISION

Name	SCHEUERKOLP, Yvette
DATE	July 21/92

EXAMINATION: ABDOMINAL ULTRASOUND

INDICATION: Liver Cyst, Elevated liver enzymes.

FINDINGS:

The previous abdominal ultrasound is not available for comparison at this time.

Diffuse increased attenuation of the liver is seen consistent with fatty infiltration.

There are several hepatic cysts. Two cysts are present in the lateral segment of the left lobe and the largest is 5.4 × 4.8 cm. A multiseptated cyst approximately 3 cm in diameter is seen in the posterior segment of the right lobe and a 3.6 cm unilocular cyst with some internal echoes is seen in the anterior right lobe.

The pancreas is poorly visualised and the gallbladder is absent. The biliary tree is not dilated.

No other abnormalities are seen.

IMPRESSION:

Fatty liver with multiple cysts.

Copy of the lab result indicating the presence of several hepatic cysts and fatty liver infiltration.

MOTHER RECEIVES A DIAGNOSIS

Towards the end of July, 1992, mother was advised that she had a "fatty liver with multiple cysts". As you can see from the copy of the lab result attached, they weren't exactly small cysts. The cysts themselves did not concern my mother too much as the surgeon who performed the gall bladder surgery had brought them to her attention. He had stated that the cysts were of no concern unless they continued to grow. Only then would they have to be dealt with, otherwise it was best to leave them alone. The surgeon had also mentioned that they were caused by my mother's prolonged use of Cafergot.

We at last knew that her fatty liver was the cause of her enlarged abdominal area. Mother asked her doctor how a fatty liver came about and how one got rid of it. The doctor said, "You eat too much". Regardless of how often my mother tried to tell her family doctor that she was not and never had been a big eater, the doctor refused to believe otherwise.

We later found out that mother's results had also showed that her liver enzymes were above the allowed range, but the doctor never disclosed this to her at the time.

* ALT (SGTP) H 52

Patient: SCHEUER KOLP, Yvette
Collection Date: 13 APR 92

DOB: 26 mar 32 ID:
AGE: 60 Y PH
SEX: F Medical

MEDICAL LABORATORIES

Patients: HRS. PC 3

TEST	FLAG	RESULT	REFERENCE RANGE	UNITS
ROUTINE CHEMISTRY:				
T. Bilirubin..............		9	(3-25)	umol/L
LD......................		271	(140-415 Paed up to 700)	U/L
AST (SGOT)		32	(0-36)	U/L
ALT (SGPT)	H	52	(LESS THAN 36)	U/L
Amylase.................		42	(LESS THAN 100)	U/L

This clearly indicates the presence of elevated liver enzymes
(liver damage). The reference range shows it should be less
than 36.

The report showed an abnormally high concentration of the enzyme ALT SGPT (serum glutamic pyruvic transaminase) in her blood, which is an indication of liver damage. The range should be less than 36, it showed at 39 in December, 1991, and at 52 in April, 1992 as you can see on the lab report. Note that this was after her gall bladder surgery. It was around that time that mother started complaining about unusual weight gain, but the doctor brushed off her complaints instead of treating them. As the doctor chose not to share the results with my mother, it led us to believe that this was a case of a physician cultivating an illness instead of curing it.

As my mother and I discussed the bad news, we decided to remain strong and get some answers. We knew for certain that a sick liver led to a dead liver, and after that the rest is history. The first step was to find out what we were up against. That meant looking up the definition of fatty liver in the medical books.

Fatty Liver: A buildup of fats in the liver. The causes include substances, as carbon tetrachloride (a clear, volatile, poisonous liquid used as a solvent in dry-cleaning fluids and in fire extinguishers), and yellow phosphorus (sometimes found in rat poisons, fertilizers, and fireworks). Fatty Liver is also seen in a nutrition disease "Kwashiorkor", caused by severe protein deficiency and found mostly in Africa, and is a rare problem of late pregnancy. The symptoms are loss of appetite, large liver, and stomach upset. The condition will usually disappear after the condition causing it is corrected or the drug causing it is no longer used.

After reading this over and over again, we wondered how on earth we could reverse this condition, because it was clear that in mother's case it was her medication that was at fault.

Drugs and their side effects –
Cafergot and Percocet:

Prolonged use of such drugs leads to problems that deplete the body in more ways than one. Some of the side effects mother experienced from Cafergot were: hot-cold flushes, sweating, nausea, diarrhea (sometimes), vomiting nervousness, itchy skin, weakness in her back, red blisters on her toes and tingling in her legs, especially at night time. Long term use also caused muscular pain and a general overall malaise. Other possible side effects include: cold skin, stomach ulcers, gangrene of hands and feet.

Cafergot (vasoconstrictor) is not intended for uninterrupted use, but mother had it prescribed to her for 15 years without ever having been made aware of its health hazards.

Side effects of Percocet (narcotic) included difficulty in breathing (later on), itchy skin, rash and mouth sores.

Although these drugs posed a great health risk, doctors chose to overlook the risk in mother's case. They even disregarded the danger to patient with kidney or liver disease.

It is important to know that withdrawal from such drugs is painful and difficult and should be done slowly.

How could she stop the medication when she increasingly needed more as time went by? We needed to find out more information about Cafergot and Percocet (Acetaminophen). We instantly headed to the nearest book store and purchased a drug-definition dictionary.

There we found more answers and were startled to read about all the side effects of mother's medication. No wonder she was plagued with all these medical problems. The odds were definitely stacked against her. Having no gall bladder, the organ which stores bile to help break down fats, was a big obstacle. Although the situation did not look promising, we kept reading.

Within a few hours we had gathered more answers than all the doctors had provided to mother in a lifetime. How, in this enlightened age, could a doctor get away with leaving his patient in such darkness? Surely mother is not just an isolated case.

That is when I began to think that my experience as a therapist, my background as a nurse's aid, and my reasonably good understanding of the medical language, might be of assistance in investigating my mother's illness. After more research I found out that the liver is the only organ capable of regenerating itself. This news provided the only ray of hope in my mother's otherwise bleak prognosis.

We still could not figure out why the doctor had not proposed any course of treatment for my mother, not even so far as referring her to a liver specialist. Was it because she knew something else and did not wish to share it? Was she (I'm sorry to say) too lazy to do her homework, or worse yet, was she totally ignorant of the situation? Whatever the reason, we were no longer interested in what could be done. We only cared about what we were going to do about it.

I became so involved in my mother's healing, that unknowingly, I absorbed more studying in a few months than I had imagined possible. I went as far as enrolling in an anatomy-physiology and medical terminology course by correspondence in the belief that other books would give me additional information. This was a long shot as far as helping my mother was concerned, but I refused to let her be subjected to ongoing medical neglect and was not going to stand by and watch her fade away.

Mother also read a great deal and our first goal was to find out how to stop the fatty liver infiltration. The obvious answer was to stop the medication which was damaging her liver. Our second goal was therefore to determine how to stop the medication when no other method of pain relief was available.

For those of you who think this was a light task, re-analyze your thoughts, because people can die from excessive pain, whether physical or emotional.

No science has yet discovered a magic pill to cure all physical sickness, or to console an inconsolable heart. With uncomplicated illnesses, doctors feel all powerful and in control. They simply prescribe or change a patient's medication leading him to believe that he is being granted a huge favour.

For many doctors, prescribing is a business and an easy consultation fee. But when the going gets tough, when more expertise is called for, they no longer want anything to do with the patient. They resort to whatever means are necessary to push the patient to the point of seeking another doctor. The patient finds another doctor only to discover that this one is no better. Doctors don't want another doctor's problem patient dumped in their lap and so they often refuse to take on that patient. Where does this leave the patient?

As I continued my research and became more confident, I was more and more determined to evaluate each and every action thoroughly and take advantage of all available resources that I could lay my hands on. It was a hell of a challenge, a challenge my mother and I met together as a team.

We concluded that in order to make a proper evaluation, she would first need to get more tests done and obtain a referral to a neurologist who might have some idea on how my mother could get off the poison that was eating away at her.

My mother went to see a neurologist. During the consultation he appeared to sympathize but ended up concluding that it was unfortunate that she had not been sent to him earlier, for then something could have been done. He went on to say that due to my mother's age and other internal problems he had no way of helping her.

Mother thanked him for his honesty, but didn't quite believe his verdict. Later on when we got our hands on her medical file, we read the following evaluation report from the neurologist to mother's G.P.:

> The patient has a bubbly personality and was seen a year ago by Dr. _____ (Pain Clinic specialist) who tried to change her medications around, but apparently the patient was not motivated enough to do so.

> The patient, however has been unable to find any other drug that will help her headaches. It seems like a fairly hopeless situation since she has in the past been tried on several different antimigraine drugs with no improvement whatsoever. He'd hope to try some other forms of therapy, including hypnosis or biofeedback (a learnable technique that enables a person to manipulate ordinarily involuntary processes, such as heartbeat and blood pressure, through concentration and knowledge (feedback) of bodily effects or responses as they occur).

> She was on Inderal and Elavil.

Reading this contradictory assessment was both frustrating and disappointing.

At first the neurologist describes mother as being bubbly, then the next thing you know he brings her down by describing her as not being motivated, which was hardly the case. Had she not been "motivated" she would never have survived the continual tragedies in her life. He then ends up agreeing that her case was hopeless because no past drugs had any effect on her.

As for the two mentioned medications, Inderal and Elavil, mother was never on those and could not figure out where he and the other doctor ever fetched them from. The one and only medication mother received at the pain clinic was a drug called Verapamil which was supposed to replace her usual medication. After taking the first pill she became sicker than a dog, felt very groggy and was in an almost zombie state of mind. This feeling lasted for three awful days. We had only looked up the drug in the drug dictionary after she took it, and to our disbelief discovered that Verapamil is used to prevent angina attacks, stabilizes irregular heartbeat, and treats high blood pressure. This drug also reduces the work that the heart must perform, reduces normal artery pressure and increases oxygen to the heart muscle. Why mother was given a heart drug, we do not know.

What we also found out going through mother's medical file, is that the doctor from the pain clinic reported having prescribed something called Fiorinal, and that mother had supposedly felt a change in her headaches and was able to control them with this medication. This report mentioned how very motivated mother was in wanting to come off her medication. That part was true, otherwise the balance of the report was totally false. She never received Fiorinal, a drug that reduces pain, fever, inflammation, anxiety and nervous tension and blocks pain messages to the brain and spinal cord. The only prescription she had ever received was the Verapamil, and you already know what happened with that one.

Believe us, people do become sick and tired of being sick, but they become even sicker when they discover, as we did, the blatantly false and negative reports exchanged by physicians. It is no wonder that some patients dont't get the required treatment, or get the wrong treatment or no treatment at all!

The medical system is in a shambles judging by the way physicians prepare their reports. If you take a minute to recall what had happened to my mother so far, it is a miracle that she managed to survive this medical negligence. On the one hand a neurologist accuses her of not being motivated enough, and on the other, a pain clinic doctor says the complete opposite. It is the back and forth exchange of such misleading information that is often the cause of mistaken diagnosis and often results in prescribing incorrect medicine to patients. Physicians win and patients lose.

However this need not continue. It is unjust for patients to have to put up with medical misjudgment which leads to improper care and unnecessary suffering. We the public must voice our concerns about those who are guilty of such faults, because it is not fair to the competent professionals to take the rap for the bad apples.

MOTHER SEES ANOTHER INTERNAL
MEDICINE SPECIALIST

It so happened that a couple of weeks after seeing the neurologist, mother saw another specialist who performed an endoscopy (a short procedure done under anaesthetic where an instrument is used to view internal parts of the body.

The following is how the specialist's report read:

Hepatic (liver) cysts appear to be simple cysts, and that the upper abdominal discomfort was probably related to pressure secondary to the cysts. It was suggested that these be aspirated.

91

Mother made no secret of the fact that she did not like that particular doctor. He was definitely the type to treat patients as though they were numbers, forgetting somewhere along the way that he was dealing with real human beings. Two weeks went by before mother returned to learn the results.

This specialist came straight to the point. He said that everything was basically normal and that the liver cysts were irrelevant (his exact word). He wanted mother to undergo an aspiration to withdraw the fluid from the cysts, which he said would ease the abdominal pressure and give him the opportunity to test the fluid as he was curious about its composition. Mother asked him if the procedure would be performed under anaesthetic and he replied "No". She asked him how the procedure was done and whether it would be painful. He clinically replied that a needle would be inserted through her abdominal cavity into the cysts and fluid suctioned out. As far as pain was concerned, there would be a certain degree of pain, but the discomfort would be of short duration. Before mother had a chance to reply, the specialist was on the phone making arrangements for the aspiration.

Mother did not wish to cut him off while he was speaking on the phone, so when he finished, she accused him of scheduling an appointment for something she had not consented to, and since he had said that the cysts were irrelevant she was choosing not to undergo the aspiration. The doctor looked furious and within seconds had seized the telephone to cancel the appointment.

Mother then asked him about her fatty liver. He rudely replied, "What do you do when you want a fat goose? You feed it". In other words, he accused her of eating too much. He then stood up, said, "Good-bye and good luck", and walked out of the room.

The following is what his report said:

She has a rather wide spectrum of deeply ingrained complaints. The first being of a big stomach which led to cosmetic surgery on her abdomen. Secondly, her dietary history is reasonably good except for the fact that it contains excessive calories. Thirdly, she denies any stress but is clearly, extremely high-strung, tense and anxious, and that her physical examination revealed a tense, anxious, overweight 60 year old white female weighing 66.4 kilos dressed.

The organs of the head and neck are grossly unremarkable. The abdomen is obese.

There are no stigmata of chronic liver disease.

This report again contained demeaning remarks and incorrect statements. Admittedly, mother did have deeply ingrained complaints, she had reason to. With all the pushing around she'd been subjected to, who wouldn't show dissatisfaction.

Mother never had cosmetic surgery because of a big stomach. She did have surgery to remove the excess skin on her lower abdomen which was the result of so many pregnancies. This procedure is commonly referred to as a "tummy tuck" and was performed in 1974. It was in no way related to mother's condition. Mother's rather extended stomach was due to the fatty liver condition and the growing liver cysts.

As far as her diet was concerned, it did not have excessive calories, if anything, it lacked sufficient calories. The doctor made an assumption without knowing the true facts.

Yes, mother denied being stressed and anxious. If she appeared high-strung, it was because she again was not getting the answers she came for.

The doctor failed to distinguish between frustration at being continually sick, and stress, anxiety and tension.

The doctor's remarks about mother's weight were unfair. She was not heavy, she had a large abdomen, not from eating too much, but from sickness.

The doctor should have reviewed his medical books before noting no stigmata of chronic liver disease. If enlarged fatty liver and steadily growing liver cysts are not indications of liver disease, then why was mother so ill?

Chapter V

Diabetes

ONSET OF RASH:

Towards the end of 1992, mother woke up one morning with strange slash-like marks around her neck area. To us, it meant that she was obviously deteriorating physically. After a big hassle, mother received a referral to a dermatologist.

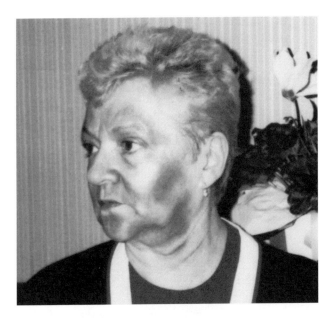

First picture taken at the end of 1992 showing mother's face rash. Little did we suspect at that point that it would not go away for a year.

The dermatologist immediately arranged for her to have a patch test, a skin test to identify allergens. No time was wasted, and within days the results came back. Both fortunately and unfortunately, the tests came back negative.

The dermatologist was intrigued because he could not pinpoint the cause of the problem and could not prescribe anything specific. Nevertheless, he prescribed an ointment that mother had used before on the multiple blisters on her toes which were caused by a reaction to Gravol. Mother had taken Gravol (prevents motion sickness, nausea, vomiting) to keep from throwing up her medication whenever the headaches reached unbearable proportions. That particular reaction was a side effect of mixing Gravol with her pain medication.

We did not know why the painful welts appeared on her neck and face. On certain days they looked as if they would go away, only to reappear with more severity. Anyone else with this condition would have been devastated, but mother insisted on going to work as usual and did not shy away from people.

Since her eyes were sensitive to sunlight, she was in the habit of wearing tinted glasses, which now served to conceal some of the rash on her face. Nevertheless she received her share of obvious stares from strangers and questions from nosy people. Sometimes she answered that she had an allergy, other times she said she had a bad sunburn.

There were a few back and forth visits to her family doctor, who was of no help whatsoever. The doctor had no clue as to what it could be and admitted that she had never in her career observed such a case. The doctor could only suggest that mother make a list of everthing she came in contact with, the type of clothes she wore, the foods she ate, the make-up and perfume she used etc. It was rather a ridiculous suggestion since the family doctor should have known by then that mother was allergic to most beauty products and did not use them. Just goes to show how inattentive and unobservant the doctor was. In the years that the doctor was my mother's family physician, she never once asked my mother to remove her tinted glasses to observe her face and eyes.

While my mother was going through another nightmare, I spent the next several months, which later turned into years, poring over reports, books and medical journals absorbing anything and everything in connection to "fatty liver" disease and allergies. I felt as though I had embarked on a new career as a medical researcher.

Mother, despite her appearance, continued to go about her daily routine as if everything was normal. We thought that maybe this latest affliction would simply disappear in time, as all the tests and all the doctors were unable to discover the cause.

As time went by, we concluded that no external factor or allergen had brought about mother's condition. It had to be the result of an internal problem. After much research, the closest answer I could come up with was that this rash resulted from long term use of medications and their possible interaction.

A drug allergy required more research on my part but at least we had something to go on. Instinctively this led us to rethink my mother's fatty liver condition and how to stop the medication which might be causing it.

IGNORED BY THE DETOX CENTRE

We called the hospital's detoxification centre and explained mother's case to the receptionist. The receptionist assured us that she would pass on our request to the doctor, who would in turn decide whether to admit my mother.

Well! Let me tell you that we were totally ignored by that center, despite our numerous attempts to get an appointment. This is what happened: on my first call, the receptionist was very receptive and told me she would call us back with an answer in the next few days. We waited a week. Thinking that maybe she misplaced our message, I called again. After a short exchange, the receptionist told me the doctor had been very busy, that she would remind him, and he would have an answer for sure within the week. We waited two weeks. I called a third time and this time was greeted in a rather hostile manner. Remaining polite, I asked the receptionist why they do not return people's calls, expecially when someone might be in critical need of treatment. She answered, "Look Miss, I passed on your messages, and he'll get back to you when his time allows". I returned, "Yeah sure! Thanks for nothing".

You bet I was angry and frustrated! Can you believe this? You call for treatment, time after time, and no one bothers to return your call. In the mean time, the sick get sicker and precious time is wasted.

The end of that year brought us nothing worth celebrating. In the New Year of 1993 mother went back to her family doctor in the hope that by seeing mother's continued state, she would take the time to help her. Her hope was futile. Again she heard, "Sorry, but it's one of those things where nothing can be done". This was not the start of a Happy New Year.

DIAGNOSIS

In May, mother received a call from her doctor's receptionist asking her to come to see the doctor for a referral to an already appointed specialist. Her latest blood-test (now routine), confirmed "Positive Hyperglycemia". In simple terms, too much glucose (sugar) in the blood.

Positive Hyperglycemia is often linked to Diabetes Mellitus, a complex disorder caused by the failure of the pancreas to release enough insulin into the body. It may also be caused by a defect in the parts of cells that accept the insulin.

> <u>Insulin</u> is a naturally occuring hormone released by the pancreas in response to increased levels of sugar in the blood. The hormone acts to regulate the metabolism of sugar and some of the process necessary for the metabolism of fats, carbohydrates, and proteins. Insulin lowers blood sugar levels and promotes transport and entry of sugar into the muscle cells and other tissues. Inadequate secretion of insulin results in hyperglycemia, and in the characteristic signs of diabetes mellitus, including lethargy and weight loss. Uncorrected severe deficiency of insulin is incompatible with life.

Upon hearing this news, mother was speechless, and so was I. Wasn't it bad enough to have life-long headaches, a deteriorating liver, and a mysterious allergy for which nothing could be done? How was mother's ailing body supposed to cope with all those ailments as well as the addition of a new one? Were we ever going to see the light at the end of the tunnel?

MOTHER CONFRONTS DIABETES

Mother and I did not give up. We continued our search for a solution. Mother went to her family doctor who told her she was scheduled to see the diabitic specialist in four week's time. Mother remarked that it was a long waiting period considering that she, the physician, seemed rather concerned about this new development. The doctor replied that she should consider herself lucky as there are only a few diabetic specialists and the first one she had called had no openings for six months.

Mother had no choice but to wait. She asked her doctor if there was anything special she should do while waiting for her appointment. The doctor replied that there was nothing except to try and avoid carbohydrates as much as possible. That didn't give mother much to go on but no other explanation was forthcoming.

Mother soon discovered that deleting carbohydrates from her diet did not leave much she could eat. Mother's favored foods included pasta, potatoes, rice and bread. She had to eliminate them as well as other products such as wieners, sausages, most luncheon meats, spreads, pates, certain cheeses, gravies, sauces..... the list goes on and on!

As it was now our habit to verify all diagnoses in our medical books, we made another important discovery. As we read more on diabetes mellitus, we were annoyed to find that the doctor had failed to mention that mother should avoid all forms of sugar. This omission on the doctor's part could have had grave consequences on mother's already fragile health.

It's a good thing mother did not have much of a sweet tooth since she also had to eliminate all sweets such as ice cream, baked products, chocolates, candies, carbonated beverages, etc. All this deprivation was very discouraging, but when living is your priority, you learn to adjust.

Mother again consulted her doctor about the allergic rash on her face and once again received a blank response.

Mother first felt numb and deserted. Anger soon followed and she had a desire to speak her mind, but being by nature a controlled person, she held it back and remained composed. The doctor gave the distinct impression that she not only wanted the disease to go away, but mother as well.

Mother came back from her consultation profoundly disillusioned about medical science. You readers are probably thinking, "Change doctors!". I say, "God knows we tried!", but none were willing to take on my mother's case. No matter which way we turned, we kept running into dead ends.

It took us a couple of days to reflect on the situation and to analyze what our options were. We were terribly frustrated about being comfronted at every turn with such an escalating and unexpected situation, which made me more determined than ever to find a solution. How soon and how fast was the challenge!

GLUCOSE TOLERANCE TEST + RESULT

In the midst of all this mother had been scheduled to take a Glucose-Tolerance Test.

> Glucose Tolerance Test: A test of the body's ability to process carbohydrates by giving a dose of glucose and then measuring the blood and urine for glucose. The patient usually eats a high carbohydrate diet for the three days before the test and fasts the night before. A fasting blood glucose is taken the next morning and then the patient drinks a 100-gram dose of glucose. Blood and urine are sampled for up to 6 hours after the dose. The test is used to assist in the diagnosis of diabetes and other disorders.

[TEST RESULT]

Collection Date   10 may 93

MEDICAL LABORATORIES
S. PC 14. CHART

DOB: 26 mar 32   ID:
AGE: 61Y   PH:
SEX: F   Medical:

ORDER: DR

2 HR GLUCOSE TOLERANCE

AMOUNT OF GLUCOSE GIVEN   75g

| | SERUM RESULTS | |
	SERUM GLUCOSE	(mmol/L) LIMITS
FASTING	9.9 H	6.1
0.5 HR	14.4 H	11.1
1 HR	17.5 H	11.1
1.5 HR	18.2 H	11.1
2 HR	19.3 H	7.8

Test result of the 2 hour glucose tolerance test. The final number stands at 19.3, way above the 7.8 limit, indicating Positive Hyperglycemia (too much sugar).

As you can see from the test copy on this page, mother's blood glucose was way above the normal limit.

Since it all had become a wait and see game, and it was evident that mother's doctor was not going to be of any help and no other physician was willing to take on mother's case, we concluded that it was time for a new approach: to go strait away to the hospital emergency should anything else occur. Perhaps we would end up with another set of doctors who would have a different opinion on mother's condition.

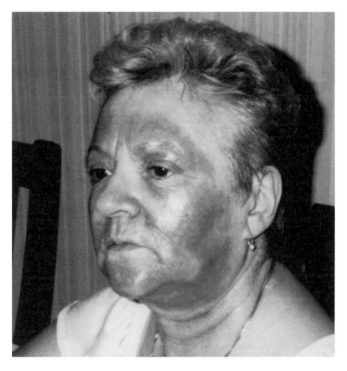

Mother's disfiguring facial rash at its worst between May and October, 1993, before receiving the Hydrocortisone 2% and only days away from our overseas vacation!

MOTHER'S FACE RASH GETS WORSE

Sooner than foreseen, on May 31st, we did end up at Emergency because mother's face worsened to a dreadful point. Upon arriving we informed the on-duty physician that mother had been diagnosed with diabetes mellitus only two and a half weeks previously.

The attending doctor turned out to be a rare exception in the sense that he was very kind, considerate, and took the necessary time to make a proper evaluation. He was of the opinion that mother was experiencing some kind of fungus infection. He prescribed a cream by the name of Ketoconazole 2%, which prevents fungi from growing and reproducing. He was almost certain that this would take care of the problem, but as a precaution he made arrangements for mother to go see another sepcialist of internal medicine.

The very next day this specialist spent an entire two hours examining and reviewing mother's condition. He did so with another female assistant, but they did not know what to make of it, and weren't sure about it being a fungus infection. They did however praise mother for holding up as well as she had considering her complex situation.

A few days of applying the cream did not ameliorate mother's facial condition, except that massive chunks of dry and hardened skin began peeling off.

MOTHER'S BODY GOES INTO SHOCK

June fourth was a day I will not soon forget. Mother was so bad that she could not even get out of bed. She told me to go to work and promissed to call me every couple of hours or so. I did not feel comfortable with the idea, but that is the way she wanted it.

Later that evening her body went into shock-like spasms. My first impression was that by the looks of things, she would not last another day. At her request I telephoned my younger brother and sister to come over for what could have been a last good-bye. God, did we cry! This could not be happening, it was just too soon.

After several more hours, I was obliged to call an ambulance because mother was in too much pain to remain at home without any intravenous treatment. She was reluctant to go, but there was no other choice.

The emergency-room doctor was one of the worst ones that we had ever encountered. Since mother was in no condition to speak, I proceeded to explain the reason for our bringing her in. His initial response was less than kind. Let's say that he was upset at my talking in medical terminology. He appeared more concerned about my speaking his language than my mother who lay suffering while waiting for treatment. I replied that I had, as he probably had done at some point, studied a lot.

Angrily he brushed my answer aside and asked why we had called an ambulance for someone suffering from some kind of headache when the ambulance might have been needed elsewhere for a more serious problem. He sarcastically told me that I should call a limousine next time. He said this before even having examined my mother. Was that rude or what?

I told him that he had wasted enough time talking to me (45 minutes) and that he should attend to my mother. He then asked what it was we wanted him to do for her?

Me: Could you please examine her, take a blood test and give her a pain killer before she passes out from the excruciating migraine headache?

Dr.: How do you know that she has such a headache?

Me: Because she told me.

Dr.: How does she know?

Me: Mother knows, and has been living with them for probably longer than you've been on this earth, and has the capacity to distinguish their differences when they occur.

Dr.: Fine, but now I need to hear it from her.

Me: (By now angry) Doctor, you've been here making continous small talk with which I'm not very impressed. Could you please stop and proceed with her treatment.

Dr.: No! I must talk to her first.

Me: Can't you see that she is in no condition to talk?

Dr.: She'll just have to manage.

Me: Why not simply take my word for it, after all, she is my mother and I know what she needs. Haven't you wasted enough time, please give her a pain killer.

Dr. Like I said, not until I've spoken to her first.

My sister and I stood looking at each other and could not believe this doctor's attitude. We observed him for the few minutes he talked with mother. When his little chit-chat ended he finally ordered a nurse to administer the pain killer she so much needed. A half hour passed and mother felt no relief whatsoever and another dose was administered. Twenty minutes later she at last felt an improvement and we were told to take her home as soon as she was able to take a few steps.

At around 3:00 o'clock in the morning we took a taxi home. We were so happy that mother had held on to dear life once again, that we determined to put the unfortunate incident at Emergency behind us.

In August, mother had another experience at Emergency, only at a different hospital. We were wrong to suppose that she would receive better treatment at a different hospital. There mother had to wait even longer because they had to repeat her blood and urine test three times before determining she had a bladder infection. The doctor had mother swallow four antibiotic pills and gave her a prescription for more which she was to take for three days.

While we sat there for six long hours, we were able to overhear the entire Emergency staff complaining to one another about having to treat more and more patients suffering from internal medical problems which should properly be treated by family physicians.

While I could understand their points of view, why did they take it out on innocent patients who had no other choice? Patients are not to blame for an inadequate system which allows doctors to push their unwanted problems onto someone else. In my view, the situation could be rectified by having a couple of internal medicine specialists on the Emergency team.

It was certainly a strange afternoon. Mother had walked into Emergency with a headache and walked out with a diagnosis of bladder infection. Later that evening she suffered a severe reaction to the antibiotics. Her face worsened to the point where it looked as if she had a third degree burn.

We were not about to return to the hospital, so we called the pharmacist. The pharmacist kindly explained to me that mother was probably allergic to sulfa, a combined form of sulphur containing antibiotics "sulfonamide" and "antimicrobials".

We waited until the next morning and went to see mother's doctor. The doctor was absent and a substitute doctor had mother undergo yet another urine test, which proved to be negative in regards to a bladder infection. To re-assure herself, the doctor ordered a copy of the hospital test from the day before, which also showed negative. It was obvious that mother had been treated for something she did not have.

By now we had had enough of these absurd medical experiences and decided to stay away from emergency-rooms and doctors as much as possible. In mother's case, each and every incident was characterized by carelessness. When you start having nightmares about going to the doctor, you realize you have to start fending for yourself.

MOTHER SEES THE DIABETIC SPECIALIST

Mother still had to face the upcoming appointment with the diabetic specialist. She did not want to go, but was curious as to what this one would have to say.

After examining mother, the diabetic specialist made the following report:

> She is a moderately obese, 61 year old female who has fasting hyperglycemia and an abnormal glucose tolerance test as well as a raised HBA1C. She has maturity onset diabetes mellitus".

His first line of treatment was to send mother to see a dietician. He was of the opinion that her diabetes was mild and that she should show a reasonably good response with a diabetic diet. If not, she would be started on an oral hypoglycemic agent. Other than that, he did not give any other specifics or any detailed instructions on what to do, except to say that she should stay away from sugars and follow the dietician's orders.

This lack of instruction was puzzling because mother was not just a patient with diabetes, she also had many other serious ailments, such as the headaches, fatty liver and face rash which no one seemed concerned about.

The diet she was requested to follow, in mother's opinion, consisted of way too much food. It prescribed three times the amount of food she was used to eating, allowing six portions of protein foods, seven starchy foods, one milk product, six fruits and vegetables, two fats and oils, plus an extra vegetable for snacks.

Mother's comment was, "How come doctors accuse me of eating too much, and here I am given more than I can chew". As this made no sense, mother kept the diet chart for ideas and modified it to her own nutritional needs. She was scheduled to see the specialist again in two months.

After she saw the specialist again, he reported:

The patient is complying with the diet given to her by the dietician, and that her diabetes should respond fairly well to it. I informed her and reassured her that the fatty liver was due to the diabetes and should improve with time.

These findings were inaccurate because the proposed diet consisted of too much food, some of which she could not eat. She was still testing foods that seemed to agree with her specific needs. If the diabetes was supposed to respond well to the diet, then why did her Hemoglobin A1C show that her fasting blood sugar level had increased by .004 grams from her previous level two months earlier?

As for the statement that the fatty liver condition was caused by the onset of diabetes, it was false as mother had been diagnosed with fatty liver infiltration long before becoming diabetic.

It's amazing how self-protective doctors can be, which is the reason why it had become so important for us to know our rights and to exercise them for our own benefit. In mother's case there was no sign of improvement, yet for some reason doctors got away with maneuvering the test results as though all of her ailments were minor.

By now all these intangibles had exhausted mother and me to a point where we decided we needed a vacation. Since mother had expressed a wish to see her brother and sisters before getting any sicker, I quickly made reservations. I thought this break would do both of us good. My research kept hitting dead ends and there weren't any medications available to heal my mother. Other medication would hide the symptoms while at the same time create other side effects, which certainly would not help her problems. Perhaps this vacation would help to clear my head so that I could start afresh upon our return.

Our trip was overseas, so chances were that mother would not pass customs because, although not contagious, her face rash looked terrible enough to be questioned. We needed something to heal her face.

We made another apointment with the dermatologist, and this time the referral was easy to get. For the last several visits to the doctor's office mother seldon saw the same doctor twice. Mother's G.P. was apparently going through a career change and was making do with substitute doctors until a permanent replacement could take over. None of the substitute doctors stayed long and therefore did not bother learning a patient's history, and usually complied with the patient's requests.

In any case, when mother saw the dermatologist, he was annoyed, not at her but at her G.P. He could not believe that he had not been contacted earlier. It had been almost a year since he had last seen mother. He was shocked to see that she had been left in such a terrible state.

He called his colleague who was equally horrified when he saw mother's face. They promised to investigate her case further and would, no matter what, find something with which to heal her face. They were pleased when mother provided them with a photograph of her face showing the allergy. They took it around to other dermatologists in their search for an answer.

They then performed a more extensive allergy patch test to make sure that nothing had been missed. While waiting for results of the patch test, I continued with my research.

THE CLASSIFICATIONS OF DIABETES

Something I had read triggered in my mind the significance of the classifications of diabetes. Each classification had different characteristics:

TYPE I: Insulin, dependent diabetes mellitus (IDDM)

TYPE II: Noninsulin, dependent diabetes mellitus (NIDDM)

TYPE III: Gestational diabetes mellitus (GDM) occurs in some women during pregnancy. It disappears after childbirth, but many women later on develop Type II

TYPE IV: Other types, includes diabetes mellitus associated with pancreatic disease, other hormonal abnormalities, side effects of drugs, or genetic defects. Patients in this class must have diabetes mellitus and one of the other diseases, (as just mentioned) syndromes, or casual factors, formerly called secondary diabetes

Now for the diagnosis:

> the beginning of diabetes mellitus is sudden in children and usually slow in Type II diabetes. The symptoms include <u>the need to urinate often, increased thirst</u>, weight loss, and increased appetite. <u>The levels of</u>
>
> <u>sugar in the blood and urine will be high</u>, the eyes, kidneys, nervous system, <u>and skin may be affected</u>. Infections are common, and hardening of the arteries often develops.
>
> (the underlined symptoms are the ones mother was afflicted with)

Finally it all began to make sense! Could it be possible that mother's face rash was due to her diabetes, and if so, why hadn't the diabetic specialist mentioned it? Surely he should have known, having examined many patients in similar situations.

Convinced that I now knew the cause of the face rash, I turned my attention to mother's swollen abdomen. As I paged through my medical dictionary I came upon a substance called Cortisone, a steroid hormone made in the liver which can also be made artificially for use in treating swelling. Was this my lucky day? I immediately looked it up in my drug book which described its uses as follows:

- Reduces inflammation caused by many different medical problems.

- Treatment for some allergic diseases, blood disorders, kidney diseases, asthma and emphysema (defect of the lung system).

- Replaces corticosteroid deficiencies.

As I continued to browse through the book, a second drug aroused my curiosity. It was Cortisol (also called hydrocortisone), a steroid hormone found naturally in the body, that reduces swelling. It comes in the form of cream, lotion, ointment and gel. It is used for "Reliev[ing] redness, swelling, itching, skin discomfort of hemorrhoids, insect bites, poison ivy, oak, sumac, soaps, cosmetics and jewelry". It also reduces inflammation by affecting enzymes that produce inflammation.

MOTHER'S FACE HEALS

Mother couldn't wait to return to the dermatologist and make our findings known to him. The results of the patch test again showed nothing, as we had expected. My mother asked the dermatologist for a prescription for hydrocortisone, which he did not refuse because the doctor had no other option to offer and it wouldn't hurt to try it. My mother asked him if her rash could possibly be related to her diabetes. He replied that he could not say for sure, but that he would look into it.

Mother wasted no time and had her prescription filled. The directions were simple enough: "Apply a small amount of the gel cream and rub it gently to the affected areas". I must say that, as with any other prescription, mother was a little frightened of the outcome. She applied the hydro-cortisone gel on the affected area of her face. About one hour later, she felt a slight sensation of heat which intensi-fied the redness on her face. We glanced at each other and thought, "Oh my gosh! Let's hope that it's not going to get worse". But in some cases, things have to get worse before getting better, so we kept our fingers crossed and went to bed.

When I woke up next morning I crept up to my mother's bed to try and have a look at her face. The room was too dark to see clearly so I had to wait until she woke up. A short while later mother woke up, went to the bathroom and with a slight hesitation turned on the light. She could hardly believe what she saw in the bathroom mirror. Except for a slight shading on the affected area, the rash had vanished. We called the dermatologist to tell him the good news. He was pleased but told us not to forget that the underlying ailment still needed to be investigated. While mother agreed with him, she was nevertheless ecstatic to be rid of the disfuguring symptom.

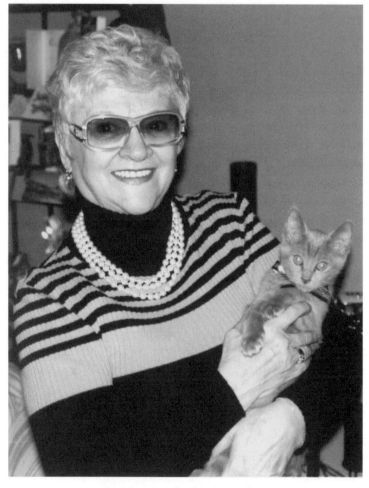

Mother as she looks today.

In October, a few days prior to departing on our holiday, mother went to see her G.P. The doctor was actually in her office that day and complimented mother on how well she looked. Mother replied, "Please doctor, do not base your judgment by the exterior of my looks because my internal problems are as of yet still unresolved". The G.P. basically ignored that comment, handed mother her usual prescription and wished her a good holiday.

Our trip was tiring, but mother was happy to have seen her brother and sisters. It was heartbreaking to see her kiss her brother and sister good-bye because neither she nor they knew if there would ever be another such trip. My mother personally considered that to have been her last trip.

A couple of weeks after our return home, she had a setback. Her abdominal area had swollen some more, so badly in fact that she literally looked pregnant. Once again she went to see the diabetic specialist who remained of the opinion that she ate too much, an opinion shared by mother's G.P. Neither doctor would do anything to help mother. It was amazing to see her carry on as well as she did, especially since her breathing had now become difficult. Her winter coat was too heavy for her to wear so we had to go out and purchase a lighter one. From an average size eight she had increased to a size fourteen (at least in her abdominal area since the rest of her looked the same). The doctors still said it was because of her diet of excessive calories. In other words, they took her for a liar.

Rather insulting, wouldn't you say? I'm sure there are quite a few people out there going though similar experiences, so my advice to you is not to give up hope. If you believe in yourself, if you follow your insticts and if you persevere in your research, you'll make a comeback.

Sadly, when certain sick people, such as my mother, happen to be able to conceal their pain and misery by being well groomed, doctors, friends and even family members tend not to believe the extent of their illness. I know of no law which says how you should look when you're sick. It's a no-win situation. Look good and no one believes you're sick, or look awful and they'll say you can't be as sick as you look. I must compliment those sick people who try to function normally when obliged to live with persistent and intense pain due to unresolved health problems.

As 1994 approached, it became more and more obvious that mother's doctors were failing to restore her health. I began to wonder if there was enough time for me to find a magical solution. Sure, I managed to develop an aptitude for self-learning, but I had yet to put my knowledge to the test.

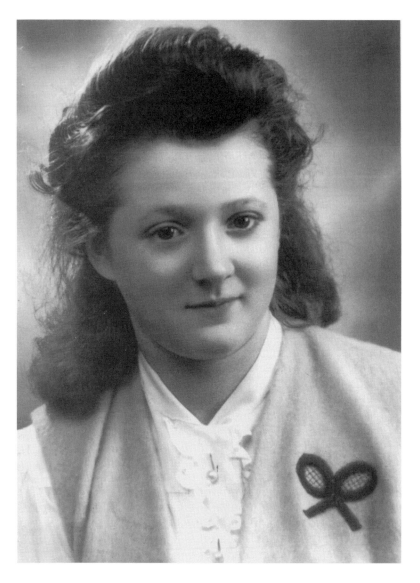

YVETTE LOUISE SCHEUER

My mother at the age of seventeen

CHAPTER VI

The Road to Alternatives

TURNING TO NATURAL REMEDIES

Mother was imprisoned in a body that suffered from numerous afflictions which hindered its performance. I knew that medications were for the most part unsafe, and were not a lasting mechanism for overcoming health problems. I therefore directed my studies towards natural remedies.

My first objective was to find something to work on her fatty liver, which I believed was the root cause of all her other troubles. Her lab results showed a high amount of serum glutamic pyoric transaminase (SGPT), which indicated liver damage. A normal level of SGPT is under 36. Mother's first lab result dated December 9, 1991 indicated SGPT at 39. Four months later in April, 1992, it was up to 52. By February 1994, it climbed to 64.

Then there was mother's hemoglobin AIC (glyocylated-hemoglobin). The normal range is 0.048 - 0.065. Mother's results were as follows:

May 12, 1993	0.078
August 12, 1993	0.082
November 17, 1993	0.079
February 10, 1994	0.109

The disturbing factor in all this was that even though mother insisted on getting copies of her lab tests and could see the results for herself, the doctors persisted in telling her that she was okay.

On a number of occasions mother asked, "Just how high and how far over the allowed range limit can one go?" The doctors would reply, "It's hard to say, becasue it's different for everybody". It was obvious that she would not get a straight answer, so she just left it at that.

No wonder people are turning towards natural healing methods. For example, garlic has always been part of mother's meals, she even increased her intake when she became so sick. She has also taken milk thistle (silymarin), which is highly recommended for all liver disorders such as jaundice and hepatitis. It contains some of the most potent liver protecting substances known. It prevents free radical damage by acting as an antioxidant, and protects the liver. It stimulates the production of new liver cells and prevents formation of damaging leukotrienes. It also protects the kidneys and is beneficial to those with psoriasis.

Mother also drank several cups per day of dandelion tea. Dandelion is a mildly bitter herb that cleanses the bloodstream and liver and increases the production of bile. It is used as a diuretic, improves function of the pancreas, spleen, stomach and kidneys. It is also taken for anemia, gout, rheumatism, jaundice, cirrhosis, hepatitis, absesses, boils, cramps, fluid retention, constipation, and breast tumors. It may aid in the prevention of breast cancer and age spots, reduces serum cholesterol and uric acid.

Mother also drank Echinacea tea. Echinacea is a bitter herb used for colic, colds, flue, infections and snake bites. It has antibiotic, antiviral and anti-inflammatory properties. It is good for the immune system, lymphatic system, and glandular swelling.

All of the above were used by mother for the last year and a half. We can't say for sure to what extent they contributed to mother's well being, but to this day we are convinced that if she had not taken them, she would never have made it. Nevertheless, we were still missing the vital ingredient and had to find it PRONTO!

MOTHER GROWS WEAKER

Day by day, mother was growing increasingly weaker and most days we had to take a taxi to work because the bus rides were no longer possible for her. It was hard to ignore the fact that she was wasting away and was being robbed of what little energy she possessed. She had begun to give me instructions regarding what her wishes were and what I should do in the event of her death. This filled me with profound melancholy and despair.

The gravity of the situation was obvious. We had to admit that in the last few days her pain was getting progressively worse and as each day went by a little more of ber body was dying. We couldn't help noticing that her weight gain was unstoppable. Her personal suffering had reached its climax. Her body was now functioning in a constant state of alarm. It was demoralizing, and for a while I felt as though I had failed and was powerless to stop the rapid advance of her medical misery.

In the last few days, mother's debilitation forced her to spend much of the time in bed, nauseous and exhausted, and we both knew that it would not be the Christmas holiday we had hoped for. We tried to pursuade ourselves that this was another unfortunate reaction caused by her multiple health problems due to medications. Drugs, whether over-the-counter or prescription, kill people. They are meant for a temporary solution to a temporary problem.

I could not stand by and watch as the disease continued to ravage mother's body and devoted my entire attention on expanding my research. I got the idea to read the complete medical dictionary from A to Z. I knew it was a long shot, but as a last resort I would have tried anything. Going through 900 pages of medical text was a monumental undertaking, but it was better than seeing someone you love wasting away before your very eyes.

I believe that the challenge of life is to try to overcome the impossible. So I plunged myself into reading page after page, definition after defition. I devoted every spare minute I had in a search for a cure. I left no stone unturned as I was not going to let the medical profession chip away at mother's pride as though she was a dispensable product of society. Medical science has forgotten the basic truth that people have value and must be respected.

Thankfully, a couple of days into my reading, I stumbled upon choline.

The miracle of choline

"Choline: A lipotropic agent, a substance that decreases liver fat content by increasing phospholipid turnover".

I immediately shared my findings with my mother and verified this substance in all of my other medical dictionaries. I went to our local library to double check my information and consumed an entire afternoon at the library verifying the validity of my material regarding the efficacy of choline. None of the library material taught me any more than what I had already learned from my own books, so my belief that books are a wise and healthy investment was reaffirmed.

Books can be like doctors: very controversial. So it is adviseable to have several manuals for research and reference purposes. You have to then decide which ones to believe using your personal instincts, that inner gut feeling, to guide you.

Now that I had the name of the substance, I still needed to get a hold of it. Not knowing whether it was available only by prescription, I reached for the phone and called the pharmacy. The pharmacist told me that it was not a pharmaceutical substance, and that I should try a vitamin store.

I was out the door and headed to the natural pharmacy. I browsed around for a few minutes until I encountered an impeccable line-up of bottles marked Phosphatidyl-Choline. I purchased one bottle at the cost of fifteen dollars and rushed back to my office to hand it over to mother. The directions were simple: "Take one to three capsules a day with or after meals". I double-checked one of my books for the ideal dosage, but the dosage varied according to the particular illness. My personal guess was to have mother take two at a time with meals, twice a day.

We could not quite believe that a simple natural substance available at practically any local vitamin store, might put an end to mother's ordeal. We were relieved however that at least we did not need the doctor's consent to obtain the choline.

I want the reader to know that we did not jump into this blindfolded. On the contrary, we were well aware that we were experimenting with something that could in all possibility backfire on us. Because mother was in such a grave and advanced stage of her illness, we felt that we had to take the chance that the choline might not produce the desired effect. When you are faced with death, you have nothing to lose by trying something new. At this point choline was the one and only hope for mother and I wasn't going to let it slip through my fingers.

December 29, 1993 was the big day. Mother waited for supper time and took the first set of two choline capsules. We sat and watched television for a couple of hours in the evening. Mother did not feel any reaction, which was a good sign as her body reacts quite quickly to any negative influences. It was also possible that mother was too sick for the choline to work on her fatty liver. Anyhow, I said to mother that it was much too soon to tell, and we would have to wait a few days before being able to judge its effectiveness.

The next morning, mother said she felt as though her breathing was easier, and that she was feeling a little less pressure in her chest area. It was a little too early to be persuaded that the choline could have acted overnight after only one dosage. I told mother that I had a simple way of finding out. When I took out a measuring tape, she looked at me and asked what I was planning to do with it. I said, "I'm going to measure your waist, or better yet, your liver area just above, since it is the biggest". I had to look twice at the measurement. Her abdomen measured 99 centimeters (39 inches). It was enormous considering her waist had always measured between 26 to 28 inches. I really wasn't exaggerating when I said she looked pregnant. I made a note of the measurement on my calendar, because that was our only method of keeping track of her progress, assuming of course that there was to be any. We had decided that she would take two cholines in the morning and two in the evening with her meals.

Hope on the horizon

On the morning of New Years Day, 1994, mother surprised me when she said that she actually felt good enough to go out for a special afternoon brunch. I immediately called the hotel for reservations and luckily they still had some space available. You can have no idea how good it was to see her for the first time in a long time enjoy a normal meal. None of us could believe the improvement over such a short period of time.

On January 6, 1994, I measured mother's abdomen again. It had come down to 96 centimeters (37.75 inches). Slowly but surely, she continued to lose her accumulated abdominal fat.

Mother's diabetes, however, showed no improvement which caused us further worry. Her February 10, 1994 test showed her hemoglobin AIC at 0.109, its highest point ever and almost double the allowable range.

MEDICAL LABORATORIES

Patient: SCHEUER KOLP, Yvette
Collection Date: 10 FEB 94

Comments: HRS. PC 13

DOB: 26 MAR 32   ID:
AGE: 61 Y   PH:
SEX: F Medical

TEST	FLAG	RESULT	REFERENCE INTERVAL
HEMOGLOBIN AIC (GLYCOSYLATED HEMOGLOBIN)	H	0.109 g/g Hb	(0.048-0.065)

NOTE: RESULT ASSUMES NORMAL RED CELL LIFE SPAN AND ABSENCE OF HEMOGLOBINOPATHY

TESTS: FBS HGBAIC

Hemoglobin AIC test result for investigating carbohydrate metabolism is obviously elevated at H 0.109. The reference range is 0.048 - 1.065.

MEDICAL LABORATORIES

Patient: SCHEUER KOLP, Yvette
Collection Date: 10 FEB 94

Comments: HRS. PC 13

DOB: 26 MAR 32   ID:
AGE: 61 Y   PH:
SEX: F Medical:

TEST	FLAG	RESULT	REFERENCE RANGE	UNITS
ROUTINE CHEMISTRY:				
Fasting Glucose. .	H	21.3	(3. 6-6. 1)	mmol/L

TESTS: FBS HGBAIC

Fasting glugose H 21.3 is almost 3 times higher than its reference range o 3.6 - 6.1.

Mother's fasting glucose was at 21.3, three times the normal range.

Mother had another scheduled blood test on February 21st, which included a routine chemistry, lipid studies, routine urinalysis, TSH, Haematology panel, auto differential. As you can see for yourself the numbers were not encouraging.

MEDICAL LABORATORIES

Patient: SCHEUER KOLP, Yvette
Collection Date: 21 FEB 94

DOB: 26 MAR 32   ID:
AGE: 61 Y   PH:
SEX: F Medical

Comments: HRS. PC 12.5, CHART
DLN: CORONARY ARTERY DISEASE OR RISK
FACTOR? NO. LDL. TRIG ALSO

TEST	FLAG	RESULT	REFERENCE RANGE	UNITS
ROUTINE CHEMISTRY:				
Fasting Glucose..	H	19.2	(3. 6-6.1)	mmol/L
Urea.		5.1	(2. 0-9. 0)	mmol/L
Creatinine		86	(30-130)	UMOL/l
Total Protein.		77	(60-80)	g/L
Alk. Phosphatase.		114	(0-125 Paed up to 470)	U/L
LD.		252	(up to 500 Paed up to 700)	U/L
AST (SGOT)		36	(0-36 Under 1 yr, up to 72)	U/L
ALT (SGPT)	H	64	(LESS THAN 36)	U/L
Gamma GT.	H	39	(Male up to 49, Fem up to 31)	U/L

Fasting glucose still high at 19.2. Liver enzymes (liver damage) increased by 12 points from the previous test.

127

LIPID STUDIES:

Cholesterol.	H	6.4	(18-30 yr Low Risk < 4.6 High Risk > 5.7	mmol/L
			31-65 yr Low Risk < 5.2 High Risk > 6.2)	
LDL (Calculated)		4.4	(18-30 yr Low Risk < 3.0 High Risk > 3.6	mmol/L
			31-65 yr Low Risk < 3.4 High Risk > 4.2)	
HDL.		1.1	(> 0.9)	mmol/L
Triglycerides		1.9	(< 2.0 12 Hr. Fasting Level) mmol/L	

ROUTINE URINALYSIS

pH.	5.0	
Protein (g/L)	Negative	
Glucose (mmol/L)	> = 55	
Ketone	TRACE	
Blood.	Negative	
Epithelial cells	Few	
WBCs/HPF	1 – 3	
RBCs/HPF	Negative	
Cast (type) LPF.	Negative	

TESTS: ESR RU UMICRO FBS TSH CHOLN SGOT SGPT ALK. PYGT LDH S. PROT BUN S. CREA HPANEL TRIG HDL

Coll. Date: 21 FEB 94Patient: SCHEUER KOLP, Yvette

* The reason for the elevated cholesterol was because of the efficacy of choline in diluting the fatty liver. It therefore produced a higher amount of cholesterol in the blood for a certain time.

Mother's cholesterol level was a little elevated. The reason for this was that choline, effective at diluting the fatty liver and other lipids, produced a higher amount of cholesterol in the blood for a certain time. This process was a cause for concern. Had we decided to increase her choline intake for faster results, it could have proven fatal as high amounts of cholesterol are very dangerous. It is always preferable to take things slower rather than risking the one chance you have by trying to hurry things along.

MOTHER'S ADVERSE REACTION TO MEDICATION:

Mother's high glucose level was a puzzle as she was following the extrememely strict diet recommended by the specialist. He told mother that since she liked to learn things the hard way, he had no choice but to put her on medication. He prescribed Diabeta 5mg 30 pk -Glyburide 5mg 30 pk. She was to take one tablet in the morning and one in the evening to lower her Glucose level.

She took only one dose and suffered an adverse reaction. She was overcome with a numb-like feeling, especially in her hands. She was unable to move her fingers or to close them into a fist, and worst of all, her now healed face had turned lobster red. I called the pharmacy and described the symptoms. The reply was immediate, "Your mother must be allergic to sulfa", and indeed she was.

Why this fact was overlooked, we never found out. We personally hadn't thought of asking. I mean, do we have to think of everything? This demonstrates once again that if patients overlook or fail to ask questions, their lives will continue to be put at risk.

First thing the following morning I called the doctor's office, explained the situation and received less than a sympathetic response. At first the diabetic specialist didn't really believe me. He was of the opinion that we were likely exaggerating the reaction. I firmly answered that it was not our intention to take up his precious time but since he had mistakenly prescribed the wrong medication, he was the one responsible for rectifying the problem. The conversation went as follows:

DR.: Your mother will have to wait until later because I'll be in meetings most of the day.

ME: But you're in the office now, can't you call our pharmacy to okay another prescription.

DR.: It doesn't work just like that, I've got to pull out her file and go over her case.

ME: How much time will that take?

DR.: Like I said, I'll get back to you later.

ME: What if she gets worse?

DR.: Don't worry, she'll be fine. Sorry but I've got to go. (hanging up)

We were sick of being continually forced to play this interminable waiting game. Did doctors take some perverse pleasure in stringing patients along? It seemed that what they were after was to have their patients completely dependent on them.

Perhaps it is true that the medical profession is consumed by a great lust for power often accompanied by wealth and therefore nature and civilized values are of only secondary concern.

In the meantime, we were again left to tackle another obstacle. We waited patiently for two days and the doctor still had not returned our call. I left a message with the doctor's secretary, who, feeling rather embarrassed, could only tell me, "He'll get back to you".

Even our pharmacist called us that day asking why we had not come back for a new prescription. We told her that the doctor was busy attending meetings. She couldn't believe it and kindly told mother to hang in there.

ABOUT CHROMIUM

Justifiably believing that we would get nowhere with the doctor, I consulted the book: "Prescription for Nutritional Healing". I read the section on diabetes mellitus which recommended chromium (GTF) supplement:

> Because it is involved in the metabolism of glucose, chromium (glucose tolerance factor or GTF) is needed for energy. It is also vital in the synthesis of cholesterol, fats, and protein. This essential mineral maintains stable blood sugar levels through proper insulin utilization in both the diabetic and the hypoglycemic. Low plasma chromium levels are an indication of coronary artery disease.

> The average American diet is chromium deficient. Research estimate that two out of every three Americans are either hypoglycemic, prehypoglycemic, or diabetic. The ability to maintain normal blood sugar levels is jeopardized by the lack of chromium in our soil and water supply, and by a diet high in refined white sugar, flour, and junk foods. Chromium is found in the following food sources: beer, brewer's yeast, brown rice, cheese, meat, and whole grains. It may also be found in dried beans, cheese, chicken, corn and corn oil, dairy products, calves liver, mushrooms, and potatoes.

Since mother was on such a restricted diet, it was quite possible that she was in fact suffering from chromium deficiency. I purchased a bottle of chromium. Mother followed the suggested dosage which was 200 mcg daily (one capsule).

Believe it or not, it wasn't until February 28th, seven days later, that we received a call from our pharmacist asking me to pick up mother's new prescription. I said, "You mean to tell me that the doctor finally called you?". She said, "No he did not. I've been so worried about your mother that I took the liberty of calling him". I thanked her gratefully for her concern and help.

The next day, in the middle of the afternoon, the doctor called to inform us that he had authorized a new prescription and that it was ready for pick- up. I could not believe his gall in taking the credit for something he did not do. I told him, "Excuse me doctor, but I do believe that it was our pharmacist who called you to okay the prescription, not the other way around. And by the way, I already picked up the prescription last night". He was not pleased with my comment, but neither were we with his attitude.

Mother's new prescription, Glucophage 500 mg – Metformin HCL 500 mg, was supposed to rectify the problem, but mother had experienced so many adverse reactions so far, that she no longer felt safe taking any kind of medication. To lessen the risk of reaction she broke the pills in half to lessen the dosage. She continued to take her daily chromium.

Mother still experienced liver cramps when taking the new diabetic pills, although not as much as with the first ones.

By March 22nd, her fasting glucose was down to 10.0, an incredible improvement in less than a month. The doctor warned her not to rejoice yet because in his opinion the level was still too high. Mother asked him why he was worrying now when he had not worried when her fasting glucose was at 21.3 not so long ago. She told him she was taking only half the prescribed dose because she felt that the chromium was helping. The doctor was upset and told her that he expected her to take the medication in its full dosage, and that her liver cramps were not related to this prescription. Mother objected, saying that they were indeed due to the pills. The doctor refused to accept her position and insisted that it was not possible (he did not want to use the words "It's your imagination", but we knew that's what he meant).

As for the chromium, he replied, "Take it or not, it won't make a stitch of difference". Mother had one last question, "What would happen if I went too low?" He answered, "Don't worry about going low, when your're diagnosed as going too high". Mother was not satisfied with his response because if her fasting glucose had come down so much in a month, the possibility of going lower was certainly there.

Ending the visit, the doctor handed mother her prescription and firmly told her that he expected her to follow his instructions. Despite his instructions, mother continued to take only half the prescribed dosage of the medication.

As April approached, mother grew increasingly tired. She had problems focusing and experienced blurred vision, all symptoms of diabetes. We agreed that she should discontinue the pills. I went to the pharmacy and purchased a glucometer, which would give mother an instant blood reading as often as she wanted.

The glucometer indicated "LO", which according to the chart meant a reading of below 2.2. Mother was right again. How was the doctor going to explain this?

We began to question just how safe one is upon entering a doctor's office. As far as mother was concerned, she had yet to receive what one could call safe and trustworthy medical advice.

Mother continued to test her blood glucose levels with the glucometer. The one thing we did know for certain was that meal times were crucially important for diabetics. It took a while to figure out a proper diet for her. Starting with breakfast at 6:30 in the morning, she had to eat something every three hours. Her last snack was at 9:30 in the evening. Depending on what her glucose level was, she ate something to bring it up down or as needed.

Her diet consisted of:

BREADS:	French bread only
DAIRY:	some cheeses (cottage cheese, cream cheese)
FRUITS:	apples pears two bananas per week
VEGETABLES:	green beans and most other beans Belgian endive with roasted garlic, parsley mushrooms red cabbage
MEATS:	chicken baby beef liver eggs one small tenderloin steak per week
FISH:	whitefish (ie. cod, sole) tuna fish (with green onions and a little moyonnaise)
BEVERAGES:	2 cups of coffee per day water orange juice (to bring glucose up) peppermint tea (to bring glucose down) fennel tea

From this selection mother chose a few foods and ate them in small portions throughout the day. After a while she was good at determining which foods her body needed and she did not need to test her glucose level as frequently.

When mother's glucose level was too low, eating a small serving of ice cream or drinking half a glass of orange juice worked best to bring the level back up. Getting that glucometer was a lifesaver. We often wondered why the doctor had never suggested it.

At a later visit mother told her diabetic specialist that she had chosen not to continue with the medication and was instead testing her blood glucose levels with the glucometer, taking chromium and following a strict diet. This angered the doctor and, looking at the glucometer, he said, "What is that thing for? It's nothing. As for the chromium, people get enough of it through the foods they eat". He told mother, "There is no need for you to see me anymore unless something goes wrong. As for anything else, your G.P. can take care of it". That was the last time mother saw him.

Mother and I had expected the doctor to have been delighted with mother's accomplishment. After all, it isn't very common to have patients come off their medication and still be able to keep their diabetes under control. On the other hand, if too many patients did as mother had done, he would not have much of a medical practice left. He was obviously more concerned with his pocket book than the well being of his patients.

As for his comment that we get enough chromium from food, he was wrong. Mother had recently picked-up a copy of the "Health Watch Canada Magazine", available free from the pharmacy. The summer 1994 issue read:

Metal Urge – The search by Canadian scientists for a leaner hog has resulted in a new way for humans to reduce stress, lower cholesterol and fight fat. Dr. David Mowat, an animal nutritionist at the University of Guelph, Ont., has discovered that chromium – an essential mineral that's required for normal glucose metabolism – reduces the effects of stress in animals. It may also contribute to leaner muscle and less fat and has helped some laboratory rats live longer. Dr. Richard Anderson, a biochemist at the United States department of Agriculture Human Nutrition Research center in Beltsville, Maryland, called that pioneering research 'a nice fit with our work' on the benefits of chromium in humans. He is convinced that chromium reduces stress and fat and helps fend off diabetes in people prone to the condition. 'The suggested safe and adequate intake is 50 to 200 micrograms of chromium,' he says. 'The normal intake is about 28 micrograms for a woman and 33 micrograms for a man.' Chromium is found in foods such as cheese, dried beans, nuts and brewers yeast. However, 'the best way to incorporate chromium into your diet,' says Anderson, 'is through a balanced multivitamin and mineral supplement'.

This article proves that some people are doing their homework! We need more such people, because the more of them there are, the stronger we will be and the healthier we will live!

All in all, things were starting to fall into place. Mother's waist had melted to ninety-two centimeters (36.25 inches), three inches less than when we started six months earlier. We were convinced that all of the natural supplements held the answers to all of mother's ailments.

That left mother's headaches, which had already lessened in frequency by about 75%.

HUNTING FOR ANOTHER G.P.

When mother's family physician called it quits to pursue another career, we had to find another G.P. Believe me, it was not easy locating a doctor that we could be content with. In mother's case the search proved even more difficult because not many doctors were willing to prescribe Percocet (a narcotic).

I called the Medical Association in our city but they were of no help whatsoever. Honestly, some of these organizations are so useless, it isn't funny!

I spent an entire afternoon calling doctors' offices in the hope that one would take mother on, but my efforts were to no avail. It wasn't until the next day, when mother went to a local walk-in clinic, that she was given a list of physicians accepting new patients. The problem with that was that you are left wondering if these doctors are taking on new patients because they are new to the block or because they are so bad that patients don't want to return to them.

One out of the twenty-nine available G.P.'s was willing to see mother. That doctor made it clear at the very first consultation that she would only prescribe the bare minimum dosage of Percocet. Mother needed two pills per day but the doctor was only willing to prescribe one and a half pills per day.

Mother had already reduced her dosage over a period of time. Her case was rather exceptional because she was able to decrease the dosage without hospitalization and/or professional help.

This doctor did not want to hear that in the last six months, mother had, on her own initiative, cut her daily dosage in half. The doctor was cold and unreceptive, and did not spare one minute more than what she felt was necessary. Mother's options were to either take what was offered or find someone else.

That visit certainly had begun on the wrong foot. Mother was never given the time to state what she came in for. The doctor insited on performing a complete gynecological exam before directing her attention to the reason for the visit. That got mother furious and she expressed her displeasure to the doctor in no uncertain terms, "I have nothing against a check-up of that kind, but how are you supposed to establish a comfortable rapport with a new doctor when you are put in this most uncomfortable position to begin with? My primary concern is my headaches, not my genitals!"

The doctor was not pleased with mother's refusal of the exam (a patient's right), and seemed to take pleasure in subjecting mother to numerous visits to show her who was the boss. Mother had to return to the doctor three times in four days just to receive 14 Percocets.

In the following five weeks, mother was obliged to make another four visits to the doctor, which were totally unnecessary since it takes only one consultation every 5 or 6 weeks for a renewal prescription.

This was by no means the first experience of its kind for mother. The same thing happened approximatley 90% of the time. Incidents of this kind occur more often than people are willing to admit.

So again we had to hunt for another physician. Let me tell you something, fighting doctors is worse than battling any disease. It is as if they take immense pleasure in reducing patients to the level of beggars. It is demeaning! While patients are struggling for mere survival, <u>the doctors of today are becoming increasingly afflicted with the selfish urges of tomorrow – unable to resist the furriest of greed, or perhaps even the hubristic temptations of science</u>.

After asking around, an acquaintance of ours was able to refer mother to someone. This doctor was so busy that he was unable to squeeze any new patients in at the time, but he did take time to talk with mother over the phone. He assured her that he would be able to see her after the summer season. Until then he would call her acting physician to work out an agreement so mother could receive the necessary medication until he could take over. Mother appreciated his gesture, but told him that calling her doctor would only create an even worse conflict. He replied that no such thing would happen.

Sure enough, on mother's next visit, her doctor did talk down to her. She did not care that the sudden reduction in Percocet would subject mother to more side effects.

If it were not for the necessity of obtaining the periodic prescriptions for Percocet and the occasional one for Cafergot, mother would seldom need the services of a doctor. I promised myself that I would continue my research until such time that doctors were no longer a necessary part of mother's life.

MOTHER'S DRAMATIC RECOVERY

Now, I'm finally able to share with all of you that mother has found a new family physician who is sympathetic to her case and is working with her, not against her. This doctor listens attentively to what mother has to say and then shares her evaluation, leading to an accord between the two of them. The days of frustration and reluctance to see a doctor are gone. Mother gets her blood tests regularly and no longer needs to beg for her medication. Mother has gone from 100 pills of Percocet she used to take in one month, down to only 30. Our objective is to eliminate them completely, which given a little more time, we are certain she will succeed in doing.

PATIENT: SCHEUER KOLP, Yvette

DATE DE COLLECTION 94/07/29 AGE 62 SEXE: F

ROUTINE HEMATOLOGY
HEMATOLOGY PANEL

WBC	9.4	(4.0 – 11.0)	GLkc/L
RBC	4.89	(3.60 – 5.30)	TErc/L
HGB	142	(115 – 160)	g/L
HCT	0.436	(0.345 – 0.465)	L/L
MCV	89	(80 – 100)	fL
PLT	198	(150 – 400)	GPlt/L

DIFFERENTIAL

Neutrophils	5.1	(1.8 – 8.0)	GLkc/L
Lymphocytes	3.7	(1.0 – 4.0)	GLkc/L
Monocytes	0.6	(0.0 – 0.8)	GLkc/L
Eosinophils	0.1	(0.9 – 0.7)	GLkc/L

GENERAL CHEMISTRY

Sodium		140	(135 – 145)	mmol/L
Potassium		4.3	(3.5 – 5.0)	mmol/L
RBS		6.1	(3.6 – 8.3)	mmol/L
Alk. Phos.		67	(< 125)	U/L
ALT	H	38	(0 – 36)	U/L
AST		25	(< 36)	U/L

RBS Taken at: 1432 h 3.0 h p.c.

INVESTIGATION OF CARBOHYDRATE METABOLISM

Hgb. AIC	0.059	(0.048 – 0.065)	g/g Hgb

Mother's ALT H 38 is almost down to normal reference range (0 - 36), all because of the supplement vitamin phosphatidyl choline. Her carbohydrate metabolism Hgb. AIC is now within the allowed range (0.048 - 0.065). Chromium supplement and a strict diet keep it under control.

Mother's last complete blood test taken July 29, 1994, showed her absolutely clear of illness. Even her ALT (liver enzymes) were only 2 points away from normal. Seeming too good to be true, mother's new G.P. agreed to have her undergo an abdominal sonogram.

ULTRASOUND

NAME: SCHEUER KOLP, Yvette
Age: 62 yrs
Dr.
Dr.
Date: Sept. 7 1994

EXAMINATION: ABDOMINAL SONOGRAM

The multiple liver cysts are unchanged in size and number from previously. The largest measures approximately 6.0 cm in diameter and is situated in the left lobe. This contains a septation.

No other intra-abdominal abnormalities are seen.

IMPRESSION: There has been no change in the number and size of the liver cysts since the previous examination.

M. D., Radiologist

Mother and I were overjoyed upon reading the result of this ultrasound report. To us it clearly indicated that we were definitely winning the battle. There is no longer any indication of fatty liver infiltration.

As you can see for yourself from the results on the previous page, there are no longer any abnormalities, and the liver cysts have stopped increasing in size. We hope that with the continuance of her natural supplements they will perhaps decalcify.

These results evidence that natural remedies are successful at healing. Mother is living proof that one can defy medical science and rectify doctors' mistakes.

Remember, that no matter what you do, keep records of all your efforts, especially keep copies of those precious laboratory results. Numbers are the most convincing evidence there is!

Mother feels like she's been born again. Her face glows as it used to do. She relishes having almost regained her lovely and petite figure.

As I am writing the last few pages of this book, I'm delighted to report that mother's waistline is down to 89 centimeters (35 inches). That's 10 centimeters (4 inches) less than one year ago. The door to a relationship is now open for her. The fears of yesterday are gone and ahead lies a future which she awaits to share with someone special.

If you have your health, then anything else is easy, depending of course on how badly you want it! I wrote this book with the purpose of presenting in a clear and concise manner, that other therapies are available for the individuals who choose to exercise their freedom of choice by treating and taking care of their own bodies with alternatives that are safe, non-toxic and very effective.

It is your right to seek treatments of your choice. Don't let yourself be intimidated by the massive medical centers full of modern technology and by the experts who disagree on which healing methods to use.

I say, who cares whether it is conventional or natural, it's what heals that counts. Our experience and knowledge became wisdom, but only after they were put to practical use. Our knowledge was in recognizing the facts, and our wisdom was in knowing what to do with the facts.

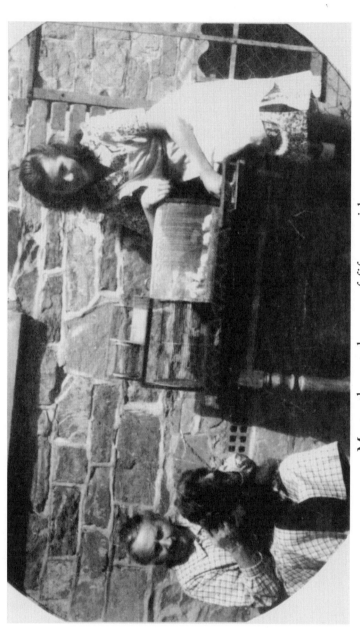

My mother at the age of fifteen with
her grandmother ANNIE NIEDERKORN.

CHAPTER VII

Vitamin Supplements

MOTHER'S REMEDIES

The following are <u>the true remedies that cured mother's fatty liver</u>:

- Two phosphatidyl choline in the morning with breakfast, followed by two more in the evening with supper for six months.

- Then two phosphatidyl choline as usual in the morning, followed by two lecithins in the evening.

(The reason for the lecithin is because of its other ingredients: Inositol, Methionine, fatty acids, Phosphate and also Choline).

- Chromium (GTF) for her diabetes.

- The coenzyme Q_{10} 60 mg daily to improve cellular oxygenation and immune function. It supplies oxygen to the liver and is a potent liver protector.

- Two capsules of Multy-zyme every morning for six months.

- One Vitamin B Complex every morning.

All the vitamins that worked for mother were taken in capsule forms (they're easier on the digestive system). The amounts she took were determined by our intuition because suggested dosages vary according to the person and the illness. In some instances you may need more, while at other times you may need less. If you are uncertain about how much to take, a vitamin consultant will help out.

We learned that the periodic blood tests were important. They served to verify if mother's vitamin intake was in the correct amount.

She survived because we had the guts to take control and the courage to place our trust in alternatives. Our decision was a smart one, and it came after mother grew tired of being shuffled from one doctor to another.

The time to think of other options is also when you can no longer count the number of pain killers it takes to ease a headache or other pain. So take charge, do what you mean to do and say what you mean to say, because one day there won't be any more days left to say and do what you meant to!

SOME USEFUL MEDICAL DEFINITIONS:
FROM BARRON'S DICTIONARY OF MEDICAL TERMS

*Thymus: Bilobed gland situated below the thyroid gland and behind the sternum (breastbone) and involved in the function of the lymphatic system and the immune system. The gland increases in size until puberty; thereafter, it becomes smaller and decreases in functional activity during adulthood.

From Dorland's Medical Dictionary:

Analgesic: An agent that relieves pain without causing loss of consciousness.

Antipyretic: Relieving or reducing fever; also, an agent that so acts.

Arachidonic Acid: A polyunsaturated essential fatty acid, $C_{19}H_{39}COOH$; a constituent of Lecithin and a source of some prostaglandins.

146

Choline: A quaternary amine, $HOCH_2$ - CH_2 N $(CH_3)_3+$, which occurs in the phospholipid "phosphatidylcholine" and the neurotransmitter acetylcholine, and is an important methyl donor in intermediary metabolism. Choline is a *Lipotropic agent, a *substance that decreases liver fat content* by increasing *phospholipid turnover. C. acetylase, c. acetyltransferase, an enzyme that brings about the synthesis of acetylcholine, c. magnesium trisalicylate, a combination of choline salicylate and magnesium salicylate, used as an antiarthritic. C. salicylate, the choline salt of salicylic acid, $C_2H_{19}NO_4$, having *analgesic, *antipyretic, and anti-inflammatory properties.

Fatty Acid: Any monobasic aliphatic acid containing only carbon, hydrogen, and oxygen, which combines with glycerin to form fat. Essential F.A., an unsaturated fatty acid that cannot be formed in the body and therefore must be provided by the diet; the most important are *Linoleic acid, Linolenic acid* and Arachidonic acid.

Linoleic Acid: A doubly unsaturated fatty acid, $C_{18}H_{32}O_2$, the most abundant such acid in various vegetable oils.

*Lipotropic: Acting on fat metabolism by hastening removal or decreasing the deposit of fat in the liver; also, an agent having such effects.

Methionine: A naturally occurring amino acid, $C_5H_{11}NO_2S$, which is an essential component of the diet, furnishing both methyl groups and sulfur necessary for normal metabolism.

Phosphate: any salt or ester of phosphoric acid.

*Phospholipid: Any lipid that contains phosphorus, including those with a glycerol backbone (phosphoglycerides and plasmalogens) or a backbone of sphingosine or a related substance (sphingomyelins). They are the major lipids in cell membranes.

FROM DORLAND'S MEDICAL DICTIONARY AND FROM PRESCRIPTION FOR NUTRITIONAL HEALING

Inositol: A cyclic sugar alcohol, $C_6H_{12}O_6$, usually referring to the most abundant isomer, myo-inositol, which is found in many plants and animal tissues. It is vital for hair growth, helps prevent hardening of the arteries and is important in Lecithin formation and fat and cholesterol metabolism. *It also helps remove fats from the liver.* It is found in fruits, vegetables, whole grains, meats, and milk. Drinking heavy amounts of caffeine may cause a shortage of inositol in the body.

FROM PRESCRIPTION FOR NUTRITIONAL HEALING

Coenzyme Q_{10}: is a vitamin like substance that resembles vitamin E, but which may be an even more powerful antioxidant. It is also called ubiquinone. There are ten common coenzyme Q_5, but coenzyme Q_{10} is the only one found in human tissue. Coenzyme Q_{10} declines with age and should be supplemented in the diet. It plays a crucial role in the effectiveness of the immune system and in the aging process. The New England Institute reports that coenzyme Q alone is effective in reducing mortality in experimental animals afflicted with tumors and leukemia.

Clinical tests are being used along with chemotherapy to reduce the side effects of the drugs. In Japan, it is used in the treatment of heart disease and high blood pressure, and is also used to enhance the immune system. Research has revealed that use of coenzyme Q_{10} benefits allergies, asthma, and respiratory disease, and it is used to treat the brain for anomalies of mental function such as those associated with schizophrenia and Alzheimer's disease. It is also benefical in aging, obesity, candidiasis, multiple sclerosis, peridontal disease, and diabetes. AIDS is a primary target for research on coenzyme Q_{10} because of its immense benefits to the immune system. Early research in Japan has shown coenzyme Q_{10} to protect the stomach lining and duodenum. It may help heal duodenal ulcers. Coenzyme Q_{10} has the ability to counter histamine and is valuable to allergy and asthma sufferers. The use of Coenzyme Q_{10} is a major step forward in the prevention and control of cancer.

Be cautious when purchasing Coenzyme Q_{10}. Not all products will offer it in its purest form. Its natural color is bright yellow and has very little taste in the powdered form. It should be kept away from heat and light. Pure Coenzyme Q_{10} will deteriorate in temperatures above 115° F.

Mackerel, salmon, and sardines contain the largest amounts of Coenzyme Q10.

No side effects have been documented to date.

The Function of Enzymes: They assist in practically all body functions. In hydrolysis, digestive enzymes break down food particles for storage in the liver or muscles. This stored energy is later converted by other enzymes for use by the body when necessary. Enzymes also utilize food ingested by the body to construct new muscle tissue, nerve cells, bone, skin, or glandular tissue. For example, one enzyme can take dietary phosphorus and convert it to bone.

These important nutrients also aid in elimination of toxins by the colon, kidneys, lungs and skin. One enzyme, for instance, initiates the formation of UREA, which is excreted in the urine, while another enables the elimination of carbon dioxide from the lungs.

In addition to its other functions, enzymes decompose poisonous hydrogen peroxide and liberate healthful oxygen from it. Iron is concentrated in the blood due to the action of enzymes, which also help the blood to coagulate in order to stop bleeding. These vital proteins promote oxidation, a process in which oxygen is united with other substances. Energy is created in the oxidation process. They also protect the blood from dangerous waste materials by converting these substances to forms that are easily eliminated by the body.

There are three types of digestive enzymes available: amylase, protease, and lipase. Amylase and protease are the two most effective digestive enzymes that are secreted in high concentrations by the human body. Amylase, found in saliva, breaks down carbohydrates, while protease found in the stomach juices, helps to digest protein. In addition, pancreatic and intestinal juices contain both enzymes. The third type of enzyme, Lipase, aids in fat digestion. Lipase is most beneficial when it is allowed to work in successive stages. Whereas pancreatic lipase digest fat in a highly alkaline environment, lipases found in food fats work in a more acidic environment.

Vitamin B Complex: The B vitamins help to maintain healthy nerves, skin, eyes, hair, <u>liver</u>, and mouth, as well as <u>muscle tone in the gastrointestinal tract</u>. B-Complex vitamins are coenzymes involved in energy production and may be useful for depression or anxiety. The B vitamins should always be taken together, but up to two to three times more of one B vitamin than another can be taken for a particular disorder.

FROM THE MOSBY MEDICAL ENCYCLOPEDIA

Choline: One of the B complex vitamins, essential for the use of fats in the body. It is a large part of the nerve signal carrier (acetylcholine). <u>It stops fats from being deposited in the liver and helps the movement of fats into the cells.</u> The richest sources of choline are liver, kidney, brains, wheat germ, brewer's yeast and egg yolk. <u>Lack of choline leads to cirrhosis of the liver</u>, resulting in bleeding stomach ulcers, damage to the kidney, high blood pressure, high blood levels of cholesterol, cholesterol deposits in blood vessels (atherosclerosis), and hardening of the arteries (arteriosclerosis). *See also *Inositol, Lecithin.*

Lecithin: Any of a group of phosphorus-rich fats common in plants and animals. Lecithins are found in the liver, nerve tissue, semen, bile and blood. They are essential for transforming fats in the body. Rich dietary sources are soybeans, egg yolk and corn. Deficiency leads to liver and kidney disorders, high serum cholesterol levels, atherosclerosis, and arteriosclerosis.

Linolenic Acid: An unsaturated fatty acid essential for normal human nutrition. It occurs in compounds of linseed and other vegetable oils.

FROM EARL MINDELL'S VITAMIN BIBLE

Methionine, choline, inositol and betaine are all lipotropics, which means <u>their prime function is to prevent abnormal or excessive accumulation of fat in the liver.</u> Lipotropics also increase the liver's production of lecithin, which keeps cholesterol more soluble, <u>detoxify the liver,</u> and increase resistance to disease by helping the thymus gland carry out its functions.

Who needs Lipotropics and why?

We all need lipotropics, some of us more than others. Anyone on a high-protein diet falls into the latter category. Methionine and choline are necessary to detoxify the amines that are byproducts of protein metabolism. Because nearly all of us consume too much fat (the average consumption in the United States is now 36 to 42 percent of total calories), and a substantial part of that is saturated fat, lipotropics are indispensable. By helping the liver produce lecithin, they're helping to keep cholesterol from forming dangerous deposit in blood vessels, lessening chances of heart attacks, arteriosclerosis, and gallstone formation as well.

'Lipotropics keep cholesterol moving safely'.

We also need lipotropics to stay healthy, since they aid the *thymus in stimulating the production of antibodies, the growth and action of phagocytes (which surround and gobble up invading viruses and microbes), and in destroying foreign or abnormal tissue.

Choline deficiency may result in cirrhosis and fatty degeneration of liver, hardening of the arteries, and possibly Alzheimer's disease.

(end of quote)

Although mother's fatty liver has healed, she will continue with her vitamin supplements, especially choline and lecithin, but on a smaller dosage (one per day). The reasons are, firstly, she no longer has a gall bladder. Secondly, for preventive and everlasting health purposes. And thirdly, because choline and lecithin keep her weight down.

The change in mother had been so visibly drastic that it was questioned by everyone who knew her. All of them thought she had gone on a diet and wanted the recipe. But honestly, there was none. It was only the choline and the lecithin that did it.

For myself and others, choline and lecithin work like magic! Since they were responsible for dissolving mother's fatty liver infiltration, it was only logical that they would also work on other body fats. In order to establish more proof, I conducted my own little experiment. We had several acquaintances and family members try the combination. After all, the only thing they could lose was a few extra pounds.

I recommended that they start slowly, first taking two cholines with breakfast or lunch for a few weeks, then taking one choline in the morning and one lecithin in the evening. I did not ask them to exercise or to cut down on food, just not to "pig out" either.

Well, surprise, surprise, it was indeed effective. The men were the most surprised when after a few weeks, their pot bellies trimmed down. All were happy with the results and are still taking their suplements today!

Starting out slowly is crucial because as you flush out the lipids (fats), your cholesterol level increases for a certain period of time. Keep a bottle of purified water close by because the program has one side effect (if it can be called that): it makes you thirsty.

We also found out that lecithin on its own produces almost the same weight loss as choline does. So to keep the weight off, taking one or two capsules of lecithin per day will suffice. Always take the capsules with food, and keep them in a cool place, but not in the refrigerator.

Life is a gift of time and our health is our greastest wealth!

Medical science holds a place in society, but it has no rules to protect the innocent victims who fall into the negligent hands of incompetent medical practitioners. Incompetence almost cost my mother her life, but in time we discovered that prevention is the key to good health.

CHAPTER VIII

The Misunderstandings between Doctors and their Patients

THE DOCTOR/PATIENT RELATIONSHIP

The following is a quote from USA Today (Sept. 1994). The comments apply equally to our Canadian emergency rooms.

Emergency Room Care *"Troubling"*

Many emergency room patients would be better off being treated by paramedics, who are likely to have more emergency care training than most doctors, a new report suggests. The preliminary report by a panel of experts, due out Monday, condemns the quality of emergency rooms, suggesting many ER doctors are *'moonlighting'* and have no training in lifesaving procedures.

'This is a very troubling segment of our health-care delivery system, one which is not really receiving adequate attention,' says Dr. Thomas Meikle, President of Josiah Macy Jr. Foundation, report sponsor.

'Doctors certified in emergency medicine fill only half of the 25,000 ER jobs. The report found many ER's staffed by:

– Other types of specialists
– Residents in training
– Doctors barely a year out of medical school

'Contrary to the public's expectations, few U.S. medical schools adequately train their students in the fundamentals of emergency care and life support,' says the report. 'Less than 20%' require courses in emergency medicine.

Dr. Thomas Bowles, president of the National Board of Medical Examiners and panel chairman, cites some of the report's recommendations:

- State Licence boards and the medical education system must ensure every medical student receives appropriate emergency room skills.

- A new classification system for ER's should indicate the level of care available, including whether doctors are specially trained and available 24 hours a day.

To put it plainly, we are faced with a severe problem in the form of an increasing sense of malaise that people experience in their doctor-patient relationship. The ever growing rate of complaints is unacceptable, it has to stop.

We have entered a stage where the lack of respect and care is becoming an ugly, degrading and evil process that will dehumanize everyone.

I believe that if we want change, it is our duty to speak our minds and make sure that our voices are heard. It may not always be the best thing for us, but it's undoubtedly the right thing to do. It is important to realize that we are all consumers of health services, and all of us have different experiences when it comes to coping with our health necessities. It is unlikely that we will all pick and choose the same methods. Whether we use conventional medicine or alternatives, questions need to be asked on both sides. We owe it to ourselves to become active participants in getting well. We should never give up hope!

People who make decisions are not perfect, yet society teaches us not to question our doctors' opinions. With all due respect to the doctors, even they do not have all the answers to the hidden secrets as well as to the inexplicable and unexpected events happening in the world. Science is failing us becasue it is not willing to recognize its own limitations. It has gained the appearance of being just another consumer product, one that makes people believe that doctors have the divine power to cure all who are sick.

Over the years, family physicians have been given too much power and now we wonder just what kind of problems they are capable of treating.

I'm very sorry to say that there is a visible decline in medical standards as well as the attention and care family physicians provide to us, their patients. A great many of us are expressing dissatisfaction but not enough of us go public. When our lives are at stake and when treatments become dangerous to our health, it becomes our duty to expose the uncooperative doctors. Gone are the times when physicians held emotional attachments towards their patients. The communication breakdown between doctors and patients needs to be rectified as it is essential to our health and well being.

The system is in a critical condition and is in urgent need of reform. It encourages a reliance on the opinions of family physicians so as to avoid an overload on the specialists. This is understandable and many of us can agree with it, but what is happening now is unacceptable.

The family doctors' approach of "one fits all recipe" should seriously be reviewed by our government. We should try to get back to the times when each ailment required its own corrective approach and when each case was assessed and treated on an individual basis. The time has come for our nation's health care providers to re-assess their values and their contributions to society. Remember that prevention is also a cure for sickness. Practicing prevention would considerably decrease the high cost of medicare. It would also help to avoid the financial drain that accompanies most medical tragedies.

DRUGS CAN BE YOUR ENEMY

For starters, do you realize that abuse of over-the-counter medicine is as hazardous to your health as abuse of prescription medicine? In the long run, all categories of drugs will cause you serious and sometimes irreparable damage due to their side effects. Drug therapy and possible addiction take an immense toll on your body and contribute to an early death. Do not abuse your immune system, for it only has a limited capacity to handle allergens and toxins which come from many sources.

Medications deal primarily with symptoms and are basically used to help control some complications, not to cure them. They are very toxic and go directly into your system, sidestepping the body's natural defenses. Most drugs interact with one another and while some have short and obvious side effects, many produce benign and chronic symptoms which are often simply accepted by the sufferer.

Doctors should make it their priority to inform their patients about eventual and inevitable complications from the continual use of medication. Too often they leave details unsaid and rely on the pharmacists to pass on some of the necessary instructions. There are no good or bad drugs, all have side effects.

You should never leave the doctor's office without the answers to your questions. (Prepare a list if you have to and don't be embarrassed about it. This way you'll save yourself another visit because of forgotten questions). Don't think that just because the doctor prescribes it, it is okay. Generally speaking, most of what doctors know about drugs is learned from the drug companies' sales representatives. Ask away, don't be shy. "Should it be taken with food or without? How many per day and at what time? Should I expect any negative reactions, and if so, what should I do? How long do I have to take these drugs and are they addictive?". Be aware that taking medication should only be a temporary solution. If you make medication a permanent companion, it will become your greatest enemy and could kill you! The choice is yours but the longer you wait, the harder it will be to avoid health problems. Do not ignore the estimated millions of lives that are placed in jeopardy and allow yourself to become another statistic.

I quote from the Oprah Winfrey show of June 23, 1994, on the subject of "Prescription Medicine", "10 million U.S. people suffer side effects from prescription drugs and 145,000 will die!"

How can numbers like that be ignored? The public has to share the blame and should be partly accountable for what is happening. After all, products would not be mass produced without markets to support them. All are guilty, the drug dealer, the drug prescriber and the drug buyer!

Prolonged and heavy use of medication can cause physical dependency with withdrawal symptoms similar to heroin withdrawal: profuse sweating, nausea, cramps, fever, body tremors and even hallucinations. Abrupt withdrawal can cause fatal convulsions.

Do not forget that we are the ones responsible for our own actions and we owe it to ourselves to stay in control and to properly maintain our health, which means avoiding getting sick in the first place. We know that environmental factors are also a problem. The air we breathe and the water we drink are filled with astonishing amounts of toxic chemicals from factory and vehicle emissions which pose many health hazards.

If it is true that human beings are the greatest of all life forms on this earth, then we are obligated to respect and protect all living creatures. We live in this world only once, but once is enough if we live our lives right. It is better to live richly than to die rich.

Maintaining your body isn't any different than taking care of your car, house or any other possession. If you wish to enjoy all of life's grand toys, for heaven's sake take care of your health first! Many health troubles can be easily avoided, for most are largely due to lifestyle.

Eliminating or at least reducing smoking, alcohol, caffeine and excess eating would be a good start. Another would be not purchasing "quick fixes" from the drug store. Just because it's advertized on television doesn't mean its okay. Do not brush aside aches and pains for they can be indicators of serious problems. Once the symptoms manifest themselves, most of the damage will already have been done and complete recovery will not always be possible.

BEING RESPONSIBLE FOR OUR HEALTH

Be aware that the health care system is not only service oriented but profit oriented as well. That is why millions of dollars are spent by drug companies on advertising in an effort to convince consumers that there is something wrong with them. When people are tired, sleepless, overweight, suffering from indigestion or what have you, is the time when they are succeptible to the claims by drug companies that their medication will solve all these problems. Unfortunately, many accept the easy way out and end up relying on pills for symptom relief instead of making the changes in their lifestyles necessary to good health.

We, the public, have to stop popping pills as if they were candies. What did our ancestors do before modern medications? Simple remedies such as garlic or homemade chicken soup may be all we need to treat colds. Many simple solutions are probably sitting in our kitchen cupboards or at our corner grocery stores. Human diseases have not changed much over the last thousand years or so, it is only that modern doctors have selected more expensive names for them.

Those who have had the good fortune to avoid encounters with illnesses should not overlook the obvious, that no one is totally immune. All will one day need medical attention and only then will they understand and sympathize with those who are in constant need. No human being wishes misery upon another (at least I'd like to think so), so take a moment to think about those victims of illness and do not take your own health for granted.

Some people appear to have forgotten to focus on being and remaining well. Is it because they believe that there is a pill to cure anything and that doctors are invincible? Doctors do have knowledge that others lack, but it is your health and your life involved so take an active role in you well being.

Today, there is too much focus on ongoing and new treatments, when in fact research should be directed towards finding preventive methods. The medical profession has lost sight of the very basic cures crucial to a society in need. Rapid advances in modern medicine have persuaded our physicians to be so obsessed with the treatment of diseases that they have forgotten that they are treating human beings.

Although year after year billions of dollars are spent on research, more and more people are developing diseases and dying from them. We are frightened by the fast rising statistics. We keep wondering "What's next? Just how bad will it get?". While statistics can be useful, they can also be a misleading guide to our nation's health. Life is a continuous learning experience and we should not allow ourselves to be intimidated by the system.

Medical professionals disagree widely on the causes of illnesses and on how they should be treated. Certain treatments fail and as a result many medical opinions may be required to determine the proper course of treatment for you. Has the time come when you have to learn how to diagnose yourself if you do not want to be depleted by never ending medical bills?

Look at the situation with our teachers. How can teachers possibly give their students the capable instruction they need and deserve when their classrooms keep increasing beyond their limits? The same thing holds true for doctors and their patients. Whether we are talking about students or patients, an overload of either will not improve our education or our health. If doctors were salaried or controlled in the number of patients they see, then perhaps this deplorable situation could be remedied.

Now ask yourself, when was the last time you had a good talk with your doctor? Did he or she really listen? The length of time allotted to a patient is a disgrace. How can there be any effective and long-lasting relationship between doctor and patient without an opportunity for communication and comprehension?

People want to be heard and it is important to them to be given a chance to express themselves. Patients are knowledgeable about their symptoms and, given time, can describe them with great accuracy, which can only help doctors in making their diagnoses. Rushed visits are extremely intimidating and unsatisfactory to patients, especially the elderly ones who may need a little time to gather their thoughts. A hurried visit may cause them to forget to mention important symptoms that could affect the course of their treatment.

LACK OF CARE FOR THE ELDERLY

No details should be overlooked if pain is to be abolished. Too many elderly people are suffering unnecessarily because physicians are largely trained to treat the young and are generally less interested in taking care of our older generation. As a result, in many instances the elderly do not receive the quality care needed.

Unfortunately, our society's attitude towards the elderly is: why care and invest time and money in someone who won't be around for much longer?

So too many elderly who could be helped are left trapped with their needs unattended to.

Frankly speaking, treatment of the elderly by our medical system is becoming a national embarrassment. We need more geriatricians to care for them, but young doctors generally avoid this field. Perhaps they have not considered that no human can avoid growing old.

Treatments are meant to vary according to an individual's symptoms and temperament, and should recognize cultural differences. But the world has not become a better place, only a more complicated one. People do not seem to have any value for one another. They are being divided rather than united. No breed of humans should be treated as being disposable. People must learn how to manage themselves and change themselves within their own entourage and make the most of the best and the least of the worst.

Anybody who thinks that money is everything has never been sick. Those who ignore health in the pursuit of wealth usually end up losing both. Why is it that our health always seems so much more valuable after we lose it?

PUBLIC HEALTH CARE – A BUSINESSLIKE PRACTICE

We no longer like what we see, but change requires leaders with a vision and a society to back them up. We know that we can't afford everything for everone, but neither do we want to deny anything to anyone. People have grown tired of all the political, economical and moral questions that have become very messy and intolerable.

When one person's health is threatened, it should become the concern of all. How can anyone think that we receive a satisfactory level of care, when all we see is medical staff stressed-out because they are now fewer in number and expected to take on more duties due to budget cuts. No wonder that there is widespread demoralization among health-care workers.

Budget cuts do not seem to have affected doctors in private practice. They see more patients and make more money. Their greed and lack of time has made some of them insensitive. They adopt an aggressive approach to convert patients to their way of thinking, and the patients who are weak get sucked into this whirlpool. No one should have to endure such business-like practices when it involves their health and their life.

We have to ask ourselves whether it is desirable to have a health-care system that pays for quantity rather than quality. I am of the opinion that when you consult a doctor, you should always reserve a tiny bit of space in the back of your mind for doubt. No one is perfect but when physicians make mistakes, patients pay with their lives. How wonderful it would be if doctors treated their patients as they do members of their own family. Maybe then we wouldn't lose so many lives. But unfortunately too many doctors still do not recognize that there is a problem, or if they do, they refuse to acknowledge it publicly.

The ups and downs of medical advisors are as capricious as the fluctuations of the stock market. How often have you as a patient been treated for one thing, only to find yourself returning to the doctor and being told something else entirely? All these flip-flops of opinions would confuse and disturb anyone.

A CASE IN POINT

As a case in point, one of my clients came to see me for treatment of excessive stiffness and limited mobility in his right shoulder caused by a fall off a ladder while cherry picking. When the accident occurred, he managed, with some difficulty, to drive home and have a neighbour take him to the hospital emergency. After the usual long waiting period, being examined and x-rayed, he was told that everything was okay except for some nasty bruising. He was given a prescription of Tylenol to control the pain and sent home.

A couple of days later he went to his family physician about the intense and persistent pain. After examining him, his doctor told him that he had suffered two broken ribs. His doctor gave him a prescription for a few pain killers and referred him to a physiotherapist. Obviously, the emergency room doctors had been negligent in diagnosing his injury. This elderly patient was subjected to the care of a group of interns who failed to see him as a human being, and regarded him only as a case study.

One's personal values can have a negative impact on others. A doctor should realize that his beliefs may conflict with the best interests of his patient. If for example, a doctor believes that his patient is overweight, lazy, and lacks self-discipline, he will project that attitude onto the patient and hinder that patient's recovery.

All of us must face "the challenge of change", and in order to meet the challenge, the medical system needs to change the way it conducts business. The change would involve restructuring of the medical industries. This restructuring should reflect the increasing need for people to work together to provide pro-active solutions in the complex interaction between doctors and patients. I hope that down the road doctors may regain pride in their abilities and the respect due them.

DOCTORS URGE ACTING CLASS IN MED. SCHOOL

The following is an excerpt from an article in the September 16, 1994 issue of USA Today:

> Doctors should take acting classes so they can at least pretend they're concerned about their patient's health, say two articles in the Lancet. Not to say doctors are cold, but the stress of medical practice sometimes spoils a compassionate mood. So knowing how to act a bit wouldn't hurt, suggest Drs. Hillel Finestone and David Conter of the University of Western Ontario.

> 'We do not put forward the idea cynically,' they say. Their concern: If a doctor doesn't have the skills 'to assess a patient's emotional needs and to display clear and effective responses....the job is not done'. They say acting classes should be required in medical school so doctors can learn just when to provide a perfectly timed compassionate look, or a touch on the hand.

> But which is better? Classical Lawrence Olivier or method acting like Marlon Brando? The doctors

hope 'comparative testing in practice' will answer that question. An accompanying commentary in the British journal by Dr. Chris McManus of St. Mary's Hospital Medical School, London, says acting may ultimately save doctors at risk of professional burnout.

Meanwhile, McManus writes, 'the surgeons, those prima donnas of medicine, hold center stage, acting out tantrums with thrown scalpels and cutting remarks'.

THE DEMISE OF VALUES IN HEALTH CARE

The following article appeared in the "Health Care News, October 1994". It was virtually impossible for me to leave it out of this book, because it confirms in large part what I have been saying about my mother's experience. Once you get people like Sister Nuala Kenny confronting the health-care crisis, then it is only logical for us consumers of services to also speak out and push for change.

The crisis in Canada's health care system is usually thought to be one of too few dollars to sustain spiraling health costs. On September 23, Sister Nuala Kenny, professor and head of the department of Pediatrics at Dalhousie University confronted the assumption that our health crisis is first and foremost a problem of money.

Kenny's lecture to over 200 participants at the St. Paul's Bioethics Conference in Vancouver was titled "Values in Jeopardy During Canadian Health Care Reform". She argued that the primary ethical and moral values that are grounded in the Canada Health Act have been virtually lost in our attempts to define the principles upon which health care reform should be based. She said that we can't afford the fancy technology that we seem to want and that 'without a fundamental restatement of values, we can't rightly, nor justly, respond to the changes that are necessary.'

Kenny is an American physician who says that she is proud to choose to practice medicine in Canada. She fears the 'rampant individual autonomy' characteristic of the United States is creeping into Canadian culture. *Health care is responding more to wants, and less to the needs of patients. It is becoming a commercial product, and physicians are falling prey to the lure of money, rather than the traditional values of the physician-patient relationship.* For example, Kenny says that the greatest moral dilemma of our health care system today is not euthanasia or reproductive technology. It is the conflict between physician self-interest and patient best-interest. She says that *physicians are out of touch with the best interests of the patient* and the value that 'scientific integrity and evidence-based medicine be firmly grounded in the physician-patient relationship.' The professionalisation of health care has expanded far beyond the scientific notion of what health care is. 'The professionalisation of health has expanded to choosing partners, getting pregnant, having a baby, raising a baby, dealing with adolescent outbreak, dealing with aging, dealing with dying, dealing with grief. And none of those are a disease.'

Indeed, problems that used to be addressed through other means are now being aggressively marketed and treated by physicians. The ultimate perversion of this phenomenon can be viewed on late night television, where hoards of opportunistic medical experts prey on insecure consumers with products guaranteed to whiten teeth, cure baldness, perfect the figure, increase mental and physical capacity, and even make house pets happier through special diets. Some medical regimens are now dangerous, irresponsible or wrong. Where will it stop?

The Canada Health Act contains several terms: comprehensiveness, universality, portability, accessibility, and public administration. Kenny says that each of these terms must be re-evaluated to determine the core value for health care reform. For example, comprehensiveness used to mean what "everything" means. Does the Canadian public deem it a priority to give liver transplants to alcoholics who have not been treated for addiction? Do we want to give new hearts to 80 year old men? *Is it reasonable to give $500 million per year to physicians who treat the common cold*, or could this become a responsibility of nurse practitioners?

There are no easy solutions or quick fixes when it comes to reforming a mammoth system that has evolved with the forces of new technologies, restructured economics and *a public who both blindly trust and despise physicians*. But Kenny's message is clear. If we only view health reform in terms of dollars, we will miss out on an opportunity to redefine what health really is, and what the values of caring are.

As you can see, the health care being provided to patients has changed considerably. It is no longer what it should be and needs a hell of a lot of change. In the meantime, everyone should work on keeping well and should become more involved in the prevention of disease rather than its cure. It in turn will make us more independent participants in our well being.

There is an urgent need to develop and improve better standards and better measures for patient satisfaction. Perhaps it will be difficult for physicians to accept change, but at some point they have to recognize the flaws and errors that are on record. We must take firm action and not place values on another's life until we understand our own values first.

CHAPTER IX

The Power of Natural Remedies your Alternative Choice

ALTERNATIVE VS. CONVENTIONAL

One of the most troubling aspects of the medical profession is that it opposes natural healing which offers alternatives to conventional medicine for the treatment of a wide variety of conditions. As I've proved to you, my mother's recovery (improvement of her damaged liver, the stabilization of her diabetes, including the elimination of medication and the decrease in the frequency and intensity of her headaches) is due to natural supplements. The effectiveness of these natural remedies is simply incredible. Where there's a will there's a way!

Through personal determination and perseverance my mother was able to attain a healthy quality of life. We now wish to contribute to the lives of others, to inspire them to not give up and to recognize that life is not measured by what we can do, but rather by the richness of our spirit and experiences. Live life carefully, for life has no spare!

The time has come to rebuild our medical system and to speak out for reform, because if we don't, doctors will likely keep their consultations relatively short and easy, and all too often will continue to prescribe medications or suggest surgeries as if no other avenues of treatment were available. If anyone so much as dares to mention natural remedies, they quickly discover that many doctors think they are just a lot of nonsense. The vast majority of doctors simply refuse to accept the fact that the natural healing process has less, if any, side effects compared to their scientific methods.

Physicians fear the media attention that the preventive approach is continuing to attract. The public is beginning to take notice of the doctors who have lost their objective to prevent, identify and treat illnesses. Respect for our medical system is declining rapidly, but we are still left with our problems. Getting an honest diagnosis from a doctor is as difficult as untangling governmental bureaucracy.

It is of great concert that the simple, sensible and safe approaches to a healthy lifestyle are almost never mentioned or put into practice by our doctors. They fail to inform their patients about other available treatment options. Most of the money spent on health-care goes to treating existing medical conditions and very little is spent on preventing them. Although many doctors don't believe that alternatives heal, I and many others think otherwise.

Most conventional physicians question the validity of an alternative view, and their arguments often sound extremely persuasive. While conventional drugs may kill the offending bacteria or hide the symptoms, the natural remedy stimulates the body's natural defences and realigns the system. Our immune system was built to respond to foreign bodies and it pays to keep it tuned. The better the state of the organism, the greater its defence.

What is regrettable is that most of us will only turn to natural healing remedies when all else has failed. People think that if it is not taught in medical school, it doesn't heal. Ask yourself, which is more toxic, natural supplements or drugs?

The alternatives are out there, but not enough of us recognize the choices we have. Our primary role as individuals should be to prevent sickness and we must have the freedom and opportunity to do so. Combining conventional medicine with alternative medicine would be an ideal solution. As the saying goes, two heads are better than one!

A good start would be for our health-care system to emphasize prevention of illnesses before extensive damage occurs. Hospitals should start leading the way in cutting costs and implementing access to preventive health care. One thing is certain, our system cannot continue as it now stands.

It is sad to have to experience tragedy or sickness before finding out who your friends are, and who the good doctors are. People are discontented and tired of being passive patients. They want to be in control of their own bodies and want to be told what is wrong with them. Surely getting an honest answer from a doctor should not be so difficult.

PREVENTION IS THE CURE

Human health requires a life-time commitment and that is why preventive methods or early detection techniques can provide the best chance for us to live full, lengthy and healthy lives. If such is our wish, and we have the desire to help reduce the exorbitant cost of health care, then we must speak-up and demand access to preventive medicine techniques.

We have grown increasingly removed from our land and its natural resources. It would be sensible to put aside our superficial way of life, and return to a more natural way of life whenever possible. We must learn to detach ourselves a bit from our fascination with technological advances. We create the culture, we set the example, and if we set a bad one, we have only ourselves to blame. As a concerned human being I'm appealing to you to "do something", before matters spin out of control.

A lasting gift to anyone, is the gift of someone's listening ear and heart, for a heart is happiest when it beats for the ones we love!

If we take the necessary steps now we can create the essential conditions for health. We are offered conventional medicine, consumer goods and services, which, in my opinion, are no more honorable than natural therapies, herbs and vitamin supplements.

Good or bad, we choose what we want and therefore it is up to us to inform ourselves prior to making a decision. We alone are responsible for our actions and our health. We mustn't forget that our bodies have amazing abilities to heal themselves, and there are numerous ways to restore them to health. So let's get going! The sooner we all learn about the vast choices we have, the sooner we can get well.

Determining the approach to treating your individual condition is the first step. In the end what counts is not what is prescribed for you, but what works for you. I do not deny that high-tech medicine can perform miracles. But if you are among the growing number of people who have been subjected to a barrage of tests and have been poked and prodded by doctors only to be told that there wasn't anything physically wrong with you, what is your alternative? If despite all your efforts to obtain relief through prescription drugs you continually find yourself feeling worse, develop additional symptoms and complications, what choice can you make?

Use your common sense and follow your instincts. This will enable you to manage the disease rather than letting it manage you. Do not allow any negative influences to distract you from your objective. Use discipline in determining what works best for you. If you are suffering, do not ignore what is happening. Once you have succeded in combating medical obstacles, it will reinforce your belief in the different healing approaches available.

CONFERENCE TOUTS PREVENTATIVE MEDICINE

Excerpt from The Health Care News – July/August 1994:

> Ten percent of The Canadian National budget, $67 billion per year, is spent on health care, making Canada the top spender for health care in the world, *but not tops in health*. This was just one of the facts introduced and discussed at the five day Partners in Care conference held at the Penticton Trade and Convention Centre last month.

> Although many concerns were raised and much was discussed during the workshops on health reform, most questions remained unanswered. 'Up to 30 percent of health care in Canada is ineffective,' (Too much money is being spent on redundant and sometimes inappropriate treatments). It was pointed out that perhaps this is, in part, because most Canadians view the health care system as an inviolate right and are apathetic when it comes to taking responsibility for their personal health and well-being.

> Of course there are a plethora of factors contributing to our $800 billion health care debt. One of the many facts presented is that *Canada is second only to the U.S. for providing the highest physician salaries, and that in Canada, physician incomes are the only health care incomes that have increased.*

For one, it illustrates that *health care has become a consumer product*. For another, it clearly shows that many people have bought into the medicine man myth: They believe that health care professionals have the divine power to cure them when they're sick, so why be responsible for their health?

It was also stressed that health care has to become less lucrative. And if most services are accessible in the community, less money will have to be funneled into large acute care hospitals that cost a lot to run and to administrate. 'The bigger the debt, the fewer the jobs'.

The bottom line is that health care has to be viewed differently by everyone in order to evolve into something financially viable and universally accessible. *And its focus should be on maintaining health rather than treating illness.*

Care givers must learn to recognize their own limitations, and only then will they become more effective healers.

In the expectation that it will result in more operational efficiency, too much time is being devoted to the integration and general coordination of medical services, and prevention of illness and the use of alternative community based services are largely ignored.

There is a need for major public education. "Prevention" means that we must educate ourselves to become more self-reliant and informed about our personal health decisions. We need to take control, avoid smoking, stay off illicit drugs, moderate alcohol intake, keep weight under control and get some form of exercise. If we don't start taking some responsibility, the end result will be inevitable for both the individual and the system. All must be prepared to fully participate. We have a stake in this, and we can make a difference.

Despite all the great accomplishments and advances of modern medical science and the most sophisticated medical equipment, we still fail to heal. If we cultivate health, there will be a lesser need to treat diseases. With proper care, the human body can stay healthy for a lifetime. If we hope to achieve a <u>real</u> cure we must learn to live in harmony with nature.

Could it be possible that science is overdosing on progress? If only researchers would focus more on preventive measures, we would have some hope that in the near future others could be spared the atrocities of pain.

In the meantime, one serious question remains to be answered: Are doctors curing illnesses, or are they cultivating them? Look at the medical treatments for cancer victims. Chemotherapy and radiation are so toxic that most of these patients are weakened to the point where their condition worsens instead of improves. Once that happens cancer treatment is often discontinued, and the patient is sent home to die. When saying yes to cancer treatment, you're also saying it's okay to kill your remaining healthy cells.

Rationally speaking, why weaken your body when you could strengthen its natural defenses with supplements, good nutrition and other natural approaches? As long as healthy cells are not damaged, they have a chance to multiply.

How many people die prematurely because of a lack of information or as a result of a wrong decision being made? Ask yourself, "Are doctors ever wrong?" Medical opinions differ from visit to visit or from doctor to doctor so that we have to wonder if the medical profession has invented a whole arsenal of syndrome diseases in order to justify the millions of dollars in prescriptions it issues each and every day.

The truth of the matter is that doctors need patients as much as patients need doctors. It would be unfair to say that medicine has no place in our society considering that it provides us with many beneficial treatments and lifesaving surgeries. But it would also be unfair to disregard nature's remedies. For many, natural formulas have proven successful where many orthodox remedies have not.

Unforturnately, natural remedies sometimes receive negative headlines in the media and people are swayed to discontiue their supplements without first verifying the facts for themselves. Rumors of quacks and con-men often come from sources with a vested interest and people allow themselves to be brainwashed into returning to conventional drug medicine.

I am convinced however that the day will come when preventive methods and natural remedies will no longer take a back seat to popular conventional methods. Natural remedies, such as nutrition, vitamins, herbs, homeopathy, and massage are shaping the ground for tomorrow's medicine! Nature heals and nature cures.

You've heard the saying: "You are what you eat". It is so true. The scenic beauty of our land is being spoiled by a variety of factors: garbage dumps, radioctive wastes, chemical pollutants, and pesticides. These contaminants find their way into our air, our food and our water. No wonder that the liver, kidneys, intestines and skin are overwhelmed. The frustrating aspect is that many people refuse to recognize and respond to what their bodies are telling them. They are off schedule with nature which is a major obstacle to good health.

You must be cautious with exercise, alcohol intake, diet and smoking. It saddens me to witness the suffering of middle-aged people trying to prove that they are as fit as younger persons. They learn in due time that the pursuit of so-called fitness later in life produces its own punishment. If they are unused to physical exercise, it could take only a few manic work-outs to cause something serious to happen. So listen to your body (it talks) and act accordingly.

We need to focus more on preventative care which means seeking our own wellness and getting to the source of our suffering, rather than relying on drug medicine which we know is not the solution. Self-responsible therapy is frequently the way to avoid expensive and frustrating care by the medical system. More and more of us are becoming aware of the problems in our food supply as well as the hazards in our environment. Substances such as dust, fumes, chemicals, and the like, invisibly present in our homes, our workplace and outdoors, can cause acute or chronic symptoms. Therefore it is to our advantage to show a greater interest in maintaining our health, and to seek recovery without the use of drugs whenever possible. Yes, recovery is possible if we have the discipline to change to a healthy diet and exercise regularly and in moderation.

As for the unresolved questions about the proper medical treatment for my mother, we've decided not to make the error of relying entirely on others, not even our doctor. We are ultimately responsible for ourselves. If we do not rely on ourselves, we would be subjected to the standards of our society, which fall short of what is needed.

It is not a question of being anti-doctor or anti-hospital, it is just that believing that you will get the best care from the medical profession is hard to do. Most of the time health care providers never seem to agree on how the quality of care should be measured and even the best of intentions get lost somewhere along the line. That is why we urgently need preventive care.

VITAMINS OR DIET?

Should you take vitamins, or simply eat well? My answer is "both". The Mosby Medical Encyclopedia has this to say:

> VITAMIN, a natural compound needed in small quantities for normal bodily functions. With few exceptions, vitamins cannot be made by the body and must be gotten from the diet or dietary supplements. No one food contains all the vitamins. Vitamin deficiency diseases produce specific symptoms usually eased by making the appropriate vitamin.

Here is a pro and con to vitamin therapy to consider:

> AVITAMINOSIS, a lack of one or more essential vitamins. It may result from lack of vitamins in the diet. It may also be the result of the inability to use the vitamins because of disease.

> HYPERVITAMINOSIS, an abnormal condition resulting from intake of dangerous amounts of one or more vitamins, especially over a long period of time. Serious effects may result from overdoses of vitamins A, D, E, or K, but rarely with the water soluble B and C vitamins.

If you take vitamins, always look for the expiration date, which shows how long the supplement should retain its potency. Vitamins break down over time so store them in a cool dry place.

Through our own experience, we have found that vitamins in capsule form are preferable to tablet form, as the capsule form is more readily absorbed and easier on the digestive tract. If used adequately and intelligently, vitamins are highly effective and relatively inexpensive.

WEATHERING THE STORMS

It was miraculous how time after time mother had managed to overcome bad medical advice. Her recovery was due in some part to her determination, but most importantly, to taking control of her own health care. Together she and I have weathered storms more fierce than either of us had ever anticipated. We won because we fought. The key to our strength was and still is the trust we have in each other.

In the summer of 1994, for the first time in her life, my mother woke up in the morning with a healthy and dazzling look upon her face.

She is now filled with an abundance of energy and is always ready to fully participate in the daily adventures of life. For me, the fear of losing her has finally vanished and has been replaced by a more tranquil outlook.

Mother's diet remains somewhat restricted and is accompanied by a little pyramid of daily natural supplements, but they are as precious as gold and are never taken for granted. They are the reason for her surprisingly rapid and unexpected recovery. We foresee that this recovery will last long enough to give her back sufficient healthy years to make up for the suffering which began the very first moment of her life.

She continues on with characteristic optimism and her outlook on life is better than ever. Recollections of her miserable days are now the only reminders of her illness.

For some strange reason, we tend to believe that our loved ones are immortal. That, of course, is an illusion, so we must thank our lucky stars when we are given a second chance. We are fortunate to love and to be loved and must not take our loved ones for granted. We must strive to hang on to that precious love for as long as we can because the loneliest place in the world is the human heart when love is absent. Love means sharing a part of ourselves with another. We do not miss what we've never had, but we sorely miss what we have lost. Life is a precious gift and love is the post powerful medicine known to mankind.

I'll stress it again: your health is an issue of prime concern, so explore your options, obtain information, and take action on the alternatives available. I hope that our example will help you make up your mind, and if it helps to save only one life, our effort will have been worthwhile.

CHAPTER X

Restoring our Culture through the Wisdom of our Forgotten Ancestors

The reason for this chapter is to illustrate that whether we deal with medicine or with society, and whether or not we like to admit it, we need to return to the knowledge of the past if we wish to heal and re-establish our culture. The past holds the secrets of tomorrow!

KNOWLEDGE OF THE PAST – THE SECRET TO TOMORROW

"For richer for poorer, for better or for worse, in sickness and in health" are words we speak and promises we make to each other. How often are these words and promises sincere? These precious vows are not only meant to be given by bride and bridegroom, they should be engraved in the mind and heart of each and every one of us. They are to be shared with the ones you love and those who are a part of your life. Love begins with honesty and life is given to us but once. When our time is up, there is no more. Life is not a play, there is no rehearsal and no encore.

Unfortunately, we have grown into a materialistic society where the elderly are pushed aside, ignored, and in some cases abandoned to face a cruel death from loneliness.

Those guilty of such conduct often feel remorse and can later be heard to say "I should have done this" or "I should have done that". My advice then is don't leave until tomorrow what you should be doing today.

We are living in an age where we cannot keep up with the incredibly fast paced society we live in. Many of us are afflicted with the "wanting too much to soon" syndrome. The reality is that with the advance of technology, almost everything is programmed and functions with the push of a button. The days of privacy are gone and have been replaced with state of the art technology and greed.

What has the world become? It is scary to think where this is all leading. Are we prepared to accept the extinction of human contact? I know I'm not. No machine and no button can ever replace human feeling, or the unique complexity of the human mind.

It is sad to see an unappreciative new generaion of people living life the easy and lazy way. They are stubbornly unwilling to admit that somewhere deep down they have not really forgotten the stories of past hardship and try to cover up their incredible guilt with a new age attitude.

To all the baby boomers out there, start facing the facts and take some time to think about what your parents and ancestors have lived through. They have witnessed the horrors of war, have endured the loss of loved ones, and have struggled with disabling disease. So stop yawning and erase that look of boredom from your face.

Yes, you have heard them recalling the same past events time and again, but is it possible that you have forgotten that learning is a two-way street? You learn from someone and in turn you are able to teach someone else. You take from someone and you give to another. Yet you seem to have the attitude that you already know it all.

Why do you want to learn things the hard way, when most everything you are experiencing today has already been experienced by your parents? Little do you know that it is in your best interest to avoid the errors of the past. How many times did you find yourself in a jam and the first thing that came to mind was to go back home for help? When worse came to worse you did not hesitate to go home and put up with your parents' endless and boring speeches. Yet when things are going well, you can't be bothered with the company of your family and are consumed by the daily rat race.

When was the last time you did something nice to show your appreciation for the endless help you received from your parents? Gratitude and love should not always be expressed with just words. Appreciation can be expressed with a simple gesture such as the giving of a little gift, taking a day off to accompany your parents on a walk, or even naming a child after one of them. Just something to show that you have paid attention and that you honestly care and respect them. You tell your children, they tell their children, and so on and so on. That is how life and memories continue after death. That is why there is and will always be such a great interest in preserving history.

You must admit that the past is most interesting and curiously intriguing. Some of you have irresistible urges to acquire and possess antiques, whether paintings, furniture, photos or other old collectibles. How these old items stir sweet memories and how you wish they could talk to you.

Yet some people cannot escape the urge to belong to this new revolutionized world which they believe offers them freedom of choice.

No one can stop the clock from ticking, but we can stop and take time to recall, collect, teach and pass on the treasures of yesterday.

Whatever you do, feel good about it and never be ashamed to show interest and to share your emotions with others whether it be laughter or tears. Tears can be of joy as well as of sadness.

Don't be unwilling to share your parents' ideas and to give them the same chance that they have so often given you. If you are one of the baby boomers, try and imagine life without modern commodities, accessibilites and opportunities. I can guess that you wouldn't know where or how to begin.

It is strange how you can make mistakes yourselves and be forgiven them, but you are not willing to accept that your parents too were entitled to make those same mistakes. Remember how they worked and struggled for endless hours and still fought to protect you and to provide you with a better future than they had. Their determination and efforts have given you what you have today which is a hell of a lot more than they themselves ever had. You should be thankful and proud that they have built roads and opened doors to give you access to endless possibilities.

To be successful you need to have a goal, no matter how big or how small it may be. I must stress that education is critical. It is never too late to continue learning. Even if you dropped-out of school, continuing education programs will give you confidence and pride. Community centers, employment offices, and such, can also help you to get started. You don't need to feel pressured or rushed, work around your schedule, a course at a time a day at a time. As you become more and more involved you will derive immense satisfaction.

If school is not your strong point, think of what you want to do and what you can do. See what is available that might best suit you. Don't be shy and don't ever feel lower than anyone else. The world is a big place and there is a spot for everyone. People need people and no one has the right to insult you or to degrade you.

The rich should not look down on the less fortunate for the rich need the services they provide. The poor should not envy the rich because often the rich have had to struggle before amassing their riches. Not everyone has the good fortune to be born into wealth and even if they have, it is not without some hardships. Becoming rich is easier than staying rich. Holding on to wealth and maintaining a privileged life demands endless hours of work.

Over the years I have had the opportunity to meet a great number of the so called rich. Let me tell you something, they work so much, so long and so hard that they are usually never at home. Most of their time is spent going from one meeting to another making deals. So yes, they sometimes do feel cranky and like to be pampered now and then. I have noticed that a great many of these people never make it past sixty-five. One wonders if they are cursed. Many of them work themselves to death. What follows is a testament, a will of succession and a distribution of the assets. A few relatives or distant family members receive a token that makes them feel happy and fortunate. Suddenly, others who are greedy and selfish, appear on the scene to demand a greater share of the booty. The one buried is quickly forgotten. It is ridiculous and quite sad.

On the other hand, compassion and love bring unity and strength which bond together and help you through the journey called life. The price of success is up to you. Always remember that the greatest reward comes from within and that is something to be aware of and to be proud of.

Think of yourself as an athlete reaching for the gold. Athletes are a special breed of people who sweat and practice hours on end, day after day, for endless years in the hopes of surpassing the feats of the ones who came before them. They strive to achieve their goal even though there is never a guarantee of success.

The overwhelming urge to succeed and the adrenaline pumping inside of you make you want to reach for the unattainable. What it all comes down to is that those willing to be patient and willing to try regardless of the obstacles in their path will become winners! It may seem that it takes forever to become a winner, but if you want it badly enough, eventually you will succeed. Sometimes, if a thing comes later and through great effort, it is appreciated more than if it comes too soon and too easily. If you plant a tree and take time to nurture it, the tree will grow strong and healthy. But if you neglect it, it will soon die.

So why is it that so many people out there don't give a damn? Could it be that perhaps our parents made one mistake, the unintentional one of wanting things to be better for us. They did not expect that in the process we would take their efforts for granted. We seem to have plenty of time for our own activities and concerns but never do we seem to have enough time available for our parents. We expect parents to remember our birthdays and special occasions, but when it comes to their birthdays or anniversaries, we somehow tend to overlook the day, or mail our wishes too late. Some never even remember to call their parents once in a while.

You are probably wondering what you should do if you don't get along with your parents? If such is the case you should come of your high horse and make the first step, or at least meet them halfway. Calmly, composedly and without angry words, try to reach some kind of compromise and iron out your differences. After all, they have given up for you, are you not prepared to give up for them or for your own children? There comes a time to grow up.

No one knows why some of us are good and some are bad, some of us healthy and some sick, some of us rich and some poor, some of us intelligent and some not overly so. You can make endless comparisons and not get anywhere. The one thing that you can do is take control of your life, be aware of what goes on around you and most of all, think long and hard before making any decision that might affect you for the rest of your life.

To simplify things, just remember this: small children – small problems, big children – big problems. You'll most likely agree that this saying applies to just about everything in life. When faced with a problem, stop waiting for it to simply go away. The sooner you deal with it the better you will feel. If you don't face the problem you will eventually find out that stress will affect you in more ways than one. Stress affects each and every one of us regardless of our economic status. No one is exempt. Some people even go so far as creating their own stress, even if there is nothing wrong with them.

Maintaining your health

Stress can be physical or mental. Not everyone handles it constructively. If it is of a short duration, you can usually cope with it. If it is a long-term thing, it will cause your body to break down. Symptoms related to stress can be digestive disorders, some ulcers, elevated blood pressure, headaches, neck aches and various others. Find a way to cope with stress. If these symptoms are not taken care of, more serious problems will arise. It is of utmost importance that you take charge of your health at once.

Physical activity may help clear your mind. It does not have to be intense exercise, a simple walk may do the trick, as long as you make it a regular habit. Hobbies are also great for relieving stress. Don't feel guilty about taking some time off or spending a little money on yourself, as your health may depend on taking measures. Don't forget your family. They also rely on you so it is important that you remain healthy.

Another very important factor is to follow a good diet and to particulary avoid junk food. You may wish to consult a dietician, or to get yourself a good book on nutrition (there are many to choose from). Another good idea is to consult a pharmacist for vitamin supplements, or to go to your local vitamin store where they will surely be able to give you some good advice. Many of these stores employ professional consultants who can advise you to the best of their knowledge.

If for some reason you still have a hard time handling stress, don't be ashamed to seek professional help. It doesn't hurt talking to someone about it. "A worry shared is a worry halved".

Another very effective treatment is massage therapy, of course. It is very natural, very healthy and extremely beneficial. But you must commit to it on a regular basis since you cannot expect your tension to disappear with just one session. Stress is an ongoing process so it stands to reason that it must be treated on a regular and continuous basis.

Take time to smell the roses, as they say, because if you don't you'll burn out long before your time. I often find myself telling my clients: "No health, no wealth", for all the money in the world is not going to cure a fatal illness.

Death is inescapable. What you can do to try to prevent it from happening prematurely is to take the necessary precautions before illness has a chance to develop and destroy you. If you think, "This is not going to happen to me", all I can say is, "It's time to wake up!"

If you consider the pace at which your life is running, chances are that you won't get to be as old as your parents. So use your time preciously, intelligently and spend some of it with your loved ones. And don't forget to put a little time aside for the elderly, your parents and grandparents. It only takes a bit of time to make someone happy but it takes an awful lot of time to rid yourself of the guilt and pain after a loved one has died.

THE GIFT OF TIME

The precious gift of time should not be wasted. It is a privilege that was meant to be invested in ourselves and in the ones closest to us. We all have a duty to protect human life as it has now become an endangered species. All of us are here for a purpose. No one knows when or why, but one day something happens, your number comes up and you are chosen to confront a situation that only you can decide the outcome of. If you are lucky, everything turns out well and there are no recriminations. If you are unlucky, all hell breaks loose and you get blamed for it.

I admire people like Mother Theresa, the Kennedys, the Princess of Wales and Bill Clinton, President of the United States. They are special because of their dedication and devotion to family unity. Yet for some strange reason the public keeps expecting unrealistic results from them. You can never please everybody but if you feel you know what should and needs to be done, come forward and show how you would solve the world's problems.

I am reminded of John F. Kennedy's address to his nation: "Ask not what your country can do for you, ask what you can do for your country". Alone, even a great leader cannot do everything for everyone. But through unity combined with courage and strength, we can make a difference.

You do not have to be rich and famous or a leader of state to be considered special. Amidst all the people of this world there are many, many special ones. We may not know them or hear of them but they are out there nonetheless and amongst them are the incredibly courageous ones, those afflicted with sickness.

Things can sometimes seem awful but there is nothing worse than when you are ill. Observe how the sick fight for each and every breath, just to live another day in the gift called life.

When my mother, my best friend, became sick, I understood why I had chosen to pursue a career in the preventive health care field. Little did I anticipate the challenges and obstacles we would have to face, but one thing I did know was that she wasn't going to give up and neither was I.

I was completely devoted and ready to confront each and every obstacle necessary to preserve and care for her for as long as life allowed and for as long as dignity remained.

One thing I do not agree with is to maintain someone on life support when there is no prospect of recovery. Life is precious, but when the time comes when it is inactive, motionless and of no value, there is no purpose in keeping a person alive. Everything we have, everthing we do is on loan to us for a certain period of time. Every human being has the right to be treated with dignity and respect. We should all support the right of individuals to make the decision to end their life.

The importance of moral values

The world is changing, sometimes for better, sometimes for worse, and humanity must regain control of it. Everything new was once something old that has been modernized. We are witnessing the collapse of tradition and the decline of moral values. I implore that we and our children have the courage to hold on to these values (e.g. family, commitment, personal responsibility, service), and to confront mistakes and correct them.

We have no defence against aging. We notice more and more that aging means feeling invisible and having to deal with discrimination when seeking new careers. Society expects the elderly to retire early and give up their desks to make room for newcomers. The younger generation is particularly unkind and inhospitable to the growing number of elders. It would be nice if we could see as they really are, not just as sick, weak and tired people.

Over the years I have met a few not so elderly pensioners, most of whom had the same complaints: "The days are long; I have nothing to occupy my time creatively; The kids seldom visit and when they do I feel as if I'm imposing".

Surely committing parents to a retirement home is unfeeling, especially when all their faculties are still functioning. You watch them dispose of all their hard earned and sentimental possessions, except for a few cherished items to remind them of their past. They shut their well-packed suitcases and close the door to the only home they have ever known and where for so many decades they lived with their memories. They proudly try to conceal their tears and go forth to meet their fate. At the last moment their greatest wish is that you have a change of heart.

Is there no way you and your parents can work it out so that with a little compromising on both sides an agreeable solution can be found? Be positive and do not forget the fabulous contributors they have been to society. Be smart and absorb the sound advice they so freely offer.

If they are healthy, they should be able to enjoy a comfortable and active retirement which can be one of the most enjoyable stages in their lives. But despite their wisdom and accomplishments, the elderly are perceived by the young as useless.

Our traditional way of life is breaking down. The rise in inequality has weakened the ties that bind families together. On occasion family life requires from us certain efforts. We must be strong and surpass the obstacles and not let ourselves be intimidated or influenced by negative outside forces.

It is my greatest wish that we all have the courage to be happy with the ones we love! To know that we are all a part of this world will give us courage. We must support social and environmental causes to keep our population safe and healthy.

We are an integral part of the natural scheme of things. We must re-establish a proper relationship with others and with nature so that together we can live in harmony. It is our obligation to put a stop to pollution and the needless destruction of nature.

So much time is spent worrying about and preparing for our future that we neglect and forget about the most important thing of all, our health. It's okay to focus on tomorrow and to look ahead, but please stop the race, slow the pace and start living! Savour every precious moment life has to offer and hold on with both hands to your dreams.

Open your heart and mind, and experience the joy that comes with sharing. Our most precious gifts, which we need most and which we cannot buy for millions of dollars, are HEALTH and LOVE.

LOVE IS THY CURE

Love is not only an amazing emotion but it is power and strength.

This poem was selected from my book of poetry entitled "The Love of Life by Viviane". Published in 1995 ©

Love is Thy Cure

Thy Love is pure
and it will endure.
Thy Love is thy future
which makes thee secure.
Thy Love is thy gain
and shall heal all thy pain.
For Love is thy strength
thy power and thy cure.

Last minute entry

June 17-1998 is a day my mother and I shall never forget.

The french edition of this book was finally a "fait accompli".

You can only imagine the happiness and excitement we felt upon seeing the finished product of our efforts. Our first priority was to phone my mother's brother "Josy" in Luxembourg to share our joy with him. What began as a celebration ended in sorrow. Just as I was about to dial Luxembourg my phone rings, it is one of our relatives calling to impart the sad and disturbing news that "Josy", my mother's only beloved brother and my dearest friend, has been tragically killed in a car accident. We were numb with disbelief. We were two shattered souls. We could no longer smile, we could only cry.

The pain of losing him is so immense, and as tragic as when mother's uncle passed away so many years ago. What adds to this pain is the fact that "Josy" was about to start writing his own book, "lack of communication amongst human kind". He had a doctorate in Sociology, an exceptional mind, a wealth of knowledge, and most of all a heart of gold. In other words, he was a man with indispensable insights he fondly wished to share.

"Josy" had been proud of my achievements, and enjoyed the thought of my helping him accomplish his long awaited dream. When death denied him of his wish, I took it upon myself to share his essence with mankind by writing this special poem in his honor, one he so richly deserves.

197

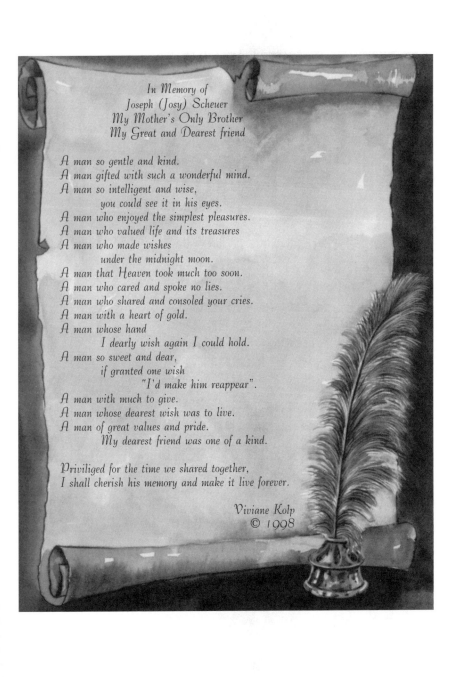

In Memory of
Joseph (Josy) Scheuer
My Mother's Only Brother
My Great and Dearest friend

A man so gentle and kind.
A man gifted with such a wonderful mind.
A man so intelligent and wise,
        you could see it in his eyes.
A man who enjoyed the simplest pleasures.
A man who valued life and its treasures
A man who made wishes
        under the midnight moon.
A man that Heaven took much too soon.
A man who cared and spoke no lies.
A man who shared and consoled your cries.
A man with a heart of gold.
A man whose hand
        I dearly wish again I could hold.
A man so sweet and dear,
        if granted one wish
                "I'd make him reappear".
A man with much to give.
A man whose dearest wish was to live.
A man of great values and pride.
        My dearest friend was one of a kind.

Priviliged for the time we shared together,
I shall cherish his memory and make it live forever.

Viviane Kolp
© 1998

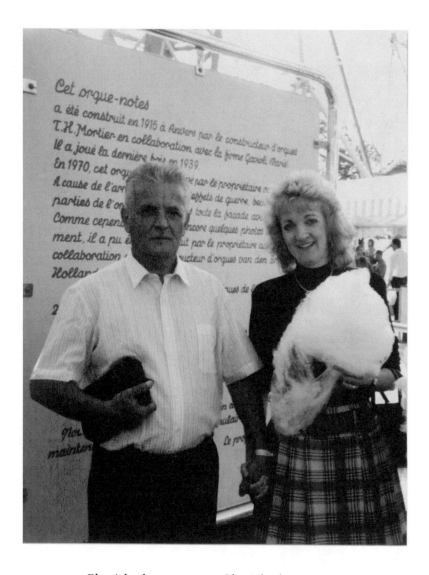

Cherished moments – Cherished memories
JOSY and ME
during a visit at the fair
in Luxembourg, september 1991

JOSEPH (JOSY) SCHEUER

March-21-1931   June-17-1998

Glossary

Albumin: a protein found in almost all animal tissues and in many plant tissues. Amounts and types of Albumin in urine, blood, and other body tissues form the basis of many laboratory tests.

Aliphatic: fatty or oily. Pertaining to a hydrocarbon that does not contain an aromatic ring.

Alk. Phosphatase: an enzyme in bone, the kidneys, the intestine, blood plasma, and teeth. It may be present in the blood serum in high levels in some diseases of the bone, liver and in some other illnesses.

Alkaline: containing more hydroxyl than hydrogen ions. The opposite of acid.

ALT, (SGPT): serum glutamic pyruvic transaminase. An enzyme normally found in large amounts in the liver. Having much more of it than normal in the blood is a sign of liver damage.

Antioxidant: a substance added to a product to prevent or delay its deterioration by the oxygen in air.

AST (SGOT): serum glutamic oxaloacetic transaminase, an enzyme found in various parts of the body, especially the heart, liver, and muscle tissue. The body makes more of it when there has been some cell damage.

Auto: a combining form referring to self.

Candidiasis: infection by fungi of the genus Candida, generally C.albicans, most commonly involving the skin, oral mucosa (thrush), respiratory tract, and vagina; rarely there is a systemic infection or endocarditis.

Carbon: a nonmetalic chemical element. Carbon occurs throughout nature as part of all living tissue and in a vast number of carbon compounds. Carbon occurs in pure form in diamonds and coal; in impure form in charcoal, coke and soot; and in carbon dioxide. Carbon is essential to the chemistry of the body. Carbon dioxide is important in the acidbase balance of the body and in controlling breathing. Carbon monoxide can be deadly if breathed in. Dusts with carbon in them can cause in many on-the-job lung diseases, as coal worker's pneumoconiosis, black lung disease, and byssinosis.

Counter: an instrument to compute numerical value; in radiology, a device for enumerating ionizing events.

Creatine: an important nitrogen compound made in the body. It combines with phosphorus to form high energy phosphate.

Creatinine: a substance formed from the making of creatine. It is common in blood, urine, and muscle tissue.

Duodenum: the first portion of the small intestine, commencing immediately after the stomach. It receives bile from the liver, food from the stomach, and juices from the pancreas.

Eosinophils: a two-lobed white blood cell (Leukocyte). Eosinophils make up 1% - 3% of the white blood cells of the body. They increase in number with allergy and some infections.

Epithelium: are cell layers covering the outside body surfaces as well as forming the lining of hollow organs (e.g., the bladder) and the passages of the respiratory, digestive, and urinary tracts.

ESR: Erythrocyte sedimentation rate, a blood test that measures the rate at which red blood cells settle out in a tube of unclotted blood. Elevated sedimentation rates indicate inflammation. ESR can indicate infection.

Ester: a compound formed from an alcohol and an acid by removal of water.

Gamma GT: glutamyl transpeptidase, an enzyme that appears in the blood of patients with several types of liver and gallbladder disorders.

Glucose: a simple sugar found in certain foods, especially fruits, and a major source of energy in human and animal body fluids.

Glycerin: a clear, colorless, syrupy liquid, $C_3H_8O_3$, used as a humectant and solvent for drugs; it is a Trihydric sugar alcohol, being the alcoholic component of fats.

Hematology: the science dealing with the morphology of blood and blood-forming tissues, and with their physiology and pathology.

HCT, Hematocrit: a measure of the number of red cells found in the blood, stated as a percentage of the total blood volume. The normal range is between 43% and 49% in men, and between 37% and 43% in women.

HDL: high density Lipoprotein. A protein in blood plasma involved in carrying cholesterol and other fats from the blood to the tissues.

HGB, Hemoglobin: the pigment in the red blood cells. It is the substance which carries oxygen to the tissues.

Histamine: a compound, found in all cells, produced by the breakdown of histidine. It is released in allergic reactions and causes widening of capillaries, decreased blood pressure, increased release of gastric juice, and tightening of smooth muscles of the bronchi and uterus.

Hydrogen: a gaseous element. It is normally a colorless, odorless, highly inflammable gas. As a part of water, hydrogen is crucial in the interaction of acids, bases, and salts in the body and in the fluid balance needed for the body to survive. Hydrogen enables water to dissolve the different substances on which the body depends, as oxygen and food substances.

Hydrolysis: the cleavage of a compound by the addition of water, the hydroxyl group being incorporated in one fragment and the hydrogen atom in the other.

Hyperglycemic: Pertaining to, characterized by, or causing hyperglycemia; an agent that increases the glucose level of the blood.

Hypoglycemic: pertaining to, characterized by, or causing hypoglycemia; an agent that lowers blood glucose levels.

Isomers: molecules with the same weight and formula but different arrangements, so that they act differently.

Ketone: any of a group of organic chemicals derived by oxidation of alcohol and containing a carbon-oxygen group. Among the ketones are acetone and acetoacetic acid.

LDL: *calculated* low density Lipoprotein.

Lipoprotein: a protein in which fats (lipids) form a part of the molecule. Practically all of the lipids in human blood are present as Lipoproteins.

MCG: microgram.

Monobasic: having but one atom of replaceable hydrogen.

Monocytes: the largest of the white blood cells. They have two to four times the diameter of a red blood cell.

Multiple Sclerosis: a progressive disease in which nerve fibers of the brain and spinal cord lose the myelin cover.

Neutrophils: granular leukocyte (white blood cell). Neutrophils are phagocytes, engulfing bacteria and cellular debris. An increase in the number of neutrophils occurs in acute infections, certain malignant neoplastic diseases, and some other disorders.

Peroxide: that oxide of any element containing more oxygen than any other; more correctly applied to compounds having such linkage as -O-O-

PH: a scale showing the levels of acid or alkaline in a solution. A PH of 7 is neutral; below 7, acid; above 7, alkaline.

Phosphorus: nonmetallic element essential in the body for calcium, protein, and glucose metabolism and for the production of adenosine triphosphate.

Potassium: metallic element, essential to life. It is the major intracellular ion, functioning in nerve and muscle activity.

Prostaglandines: one of several strong hormonelike fatty acids that acts in small amounts on certain organs. They are made in tiny amounts and have many different effects. Prostaglandines given by nasal spray, in tablets, or dissolved in liquids cause changes in smooth muscle tone, hormone functions, and in the autonomic and central nervous systems. Prostaglandines are used to end pregnancy and to treat asthma and too much stomach acid.

Protein: any of a group of organic compounds composed of one or more chains of amino acids and forming an essential part of all living organisms.

RBC: red blood cell.

Sodium: a soft grayish and metallic element needed in small amounts for health. It is eaten in the form of salt.

TSH: thyroid stimulating hormone.

Ubiquinone: a group of quinones occurring in the lipid core of inner mitochondrial membranes and functioning in electron transfer reactions.

Unsaturated Fatty Acid: fatty acid in which some of the atoms are joined by double or triple valence bonds that are easily split, enabling other substances to join to them. Monounsaturated fatty acids, found in olive oil, chicken, almonds, and some other nuts, have one double or triple bond per molecule. Polyunsaturated fatty acids, found in fish, corn, and soybean and safflower oil, have more than one double or triple bond per molecule. A diet high in polyunsaturated fatty acids and low in saturated fatty acids has been linked in some studies to low serum cholesterol levels.

Urea: 1) main breakdown product of proteins and the form in which nitrogen is excreted from the body in the urine. 2) Diuretic preparation used to reduce cerebrospinal and intraocular fluid pressure.

WBC: white blood cell.

Bibliography

The following listed books are the ones I used for my research.

Prescription For Nutritional Healing
A practical A - Z reference to drug-free remedies using vitamins, minerals, herb and food supplements. Highly recommended.
By   James F. Balch, M.D.,
      Phyllis A. Balch, C.N.C.

Complete Guide to Prescription and Non-Prescription Drugs
By   H. Winter Griffith, M.D.
      – 6th edition

The Mosby Medical Encyclopedia
By   Walter D. Glanze (managing editor)
      Kenneth N. Anderson (editor and medical writer)
      Lois E. Anderson (consulting editor and writer)

Barron's Dictionary of Medical Terms For the Nonmedical Person
By   Mikel A. Rothenberg, M.D.
      Charles F. Chapman
      – second edition

Dorland's Pocket Medical Dictionary
By   W.B. Saunders Company

Earl Mindell's Vitamin Bible

The Pocket Oxford Dictionary of Current English

The New American Medical Dictionary and Health Manual
By   Robert E. Rothenberg, M.D., F.A.C.S.